DOCTOR

BOOK TWO

ITV Books

DOCTOR

BOOK TWO

DR KEN DICKINSON

MB ChB FRCGP

The Editor wishes to thank John Oxley and the production team of the ATV series.

Editor: John Doyle
Assistant Editor: Jane Struthers
Designer: Jeremy Dixon

INDEPENDENT TELEVISION BOOKS LTD
247 Tottenham Court Road, London W1P 0AU

First published 1981

© Text, Dr Ken Dickinson MB ChB FRCGP 1981

© Doctor, ATV Network Ltd 1981

© Illustrations, ITV Books 1981

ISBN: 0 900727 88 8

Set in 10/11pt Times Roman by The Yale Press Ltd

CONDITIONS OF SALE

Illustrations by Howard Prescott

Printed in Great Britain by Whitstable Litho Ltd, Millstrood Road, Whitstable, Kent

Biography

Dr Ken Dickinson is University Medical Officer at Birmingham, where he qualified in 1961. Before this, he was in single-handed general practice for 12 years. He has always taken a keen interest in psychiatry and medical education, and recently took a three-month course in occupational health, at the London School of Hygiene and Tropical Medicine. His love of open spaces has taken him once to Newfoundland, and three times to the Himalayas, as medical officer to various expeditions. In the future, he hopes to continue his explorations as far as the Andes and the Far East.

Contents

Contents

Introduction

There are about 25,000 general practitioners in this country. The number of patients seen by such doctors varies considerably, according to several factors. Is the practice large or small? In the town or country? Are there many young children or old people? What is the time of year? Is there a minor epidemic of whooping cough or influenza?

Some doctors always seem to be busy and others always seem to have time for a chat, but none of us seem to have enough time to discuss your problems with you as fully as you would like. So, quite rightly, you look elsewhere for more detailed knowledge. One result of this is the third series of the ATV programme 'Doctor', which attempts to deal with a further selection of fairly common medical problems in a sensible, practical, realistic way.

Don't forget that the programmes you see, and the chapters in this book, are brief accounts of complex problems. They do not attempt to cover in depth the subjects discussed. They are guidelines to help you, but you should consult your own general practitioner for the specific diagnosis and treatment of any condition troubling you.

Please also remember that medicine is an art as well as a science, and that there is still much that we do not know. Also, unfortunately, much that we think we know now will be proved incorrect sooner or later. I must accept responsibility for this book and hope that most of it will remain factual for a long time. I hope that you find in it a reasonable and balanced account of the conditions described. If, after reading it, you are at least determined to stop smoking, I shall be delighted. If, as well, you remembered always to wear a safety belt in a car, keep your weight down and exercise on a regular basis, the numbers attending doctors' surgeries would certainly drop and we would have more time to talk to you!

Unfortunately, I cannot enter into any correspondence about medical problems.

Dr Ken Dickinson, 1981

Epilepsy

The word *epilepsy*, or the knowledge that somebody you know and love is subject to *fits*, is frightening and invariably causes considerable worry. I hope to show in this chapter that although epilepsy can be a serious problem, the labelling of a person as epileptic is often unfortunate, unfair and can in many cases lead to him being condemned to an unnecessarily restricted life. Epilepsy is the name given to a group of conditions, ranging from a minimal change, such as a brief stop in conversation and an eye blink, to a total loss of consciousness with muscle spasm and rigidity, which can last for some minutes.

What is epilepsy?

Basically, epilepsy is a disruption of normal brain activity. Think of the brain as an enormous computer, with electric currents flowing between millions of terminals. The interaction of this vast network enables one to think, feel and act. If the electrical activity in certain parts of the brain is disrupted, epilepsy can result. That may sound somewhat long-winded but it is often extremely difficult in medicine to give a simple definition in one sentence. Therefore I think it would be better if I move on and describe some of the characteristics of various types of epilepsy. This definition may then seem clearer.

Incidence
Epilepsy is a relatively common disorder. It is estimated that about five in every thousand people suffer from it and that in Great Britain there are 300,000 diagnosed cases. Usually, it first appears in childhood, but cases which occur for the first time in patients over the age of 30 are likely to be investigated much more carefully by clinics. It is certain that there is some hereditary element in epilepsy. If one or both parents has a history of epilepsy, the cause of which is unknown, the incidence of the condition in their children will be about 5%.

Infantile convulsions

The first attack can occur at a very young age indeed, but at the same time, because a young baby suffers from a *convulsion*, it does not mean that the baby is going to suffer from repeated convulsions or fits thereafter. Very often, children under the age of about two who suffer from a very high temperature have what is known as a *febrile* or *infantile convulsion*. The child is hot, sweaty and uncomfortable, then suddenly loses consciousness, and the limbs turn rigid before going into spasm. Naturally, the parents are extremely worried, and summon their doctor at once. However, almost invariably by the time he has arrived, the whole incident is over, leaving the child still hot, listless and drowsy, or deeply asleep.

What has happened is that the high temperature has triggered off an electrical discharge which has disrupted the brain activity, and produced a form of fit which is identical to true epilepsy. However, because it only happens to young children running a high temperature it is not true epilepsy and will not persist into adult life.

The simplest way of dealing with this problem is to stop young children from producing high temperatures, and this can easily be done at home. Any young child suffering from a high temperature should be sponged down with lukewarm water, or given a tepid bath. The effect on the child is dramatic. He feels much more comfortable and relaxed, and if the child is dried carefully in a large towel, dressed in clean pyjamas and put back to bed, with fresh sheets, he will settle well for the next few hours. There is no doubt that sometimes when looking after young children one may have to do this two or three times a night. To my mind it is well worth it, and having seen two of my children have convulsions I would certainly follow this procedure again if I thought it necessary. It is, of course, beneficial if there is no risk of the child having a fit, because it will relieve the discomfort of a high temperature.

Epileptic fits

The brief description just given of an infantile convulsion also applies to a major, or *grand mal*, attack. The patient often has a preliminary odd sensation, which warns him that an epileptic attack is about to start. This warning period is usually quite brief. Following this, the patient loses consciousness and, if standing, will fall to the ground. The patient becomes rigid, and the spasm of the breathing muscles produces a sudden outpushing of air, giving rise to a sound or a cry. This phase of rigidity lasts between 20 and 30 seconds, during which time the patient is unable to breathe, and the face gradually turns blue. The next phase, which also lasts about 30 seconds, consists of forceful, strong jerking movements of the face, body and limbs. The movements of the jaw and mouth cause saliva to froth out, making the patient appear to be in very considerable stress. After this all movements cease, and the patient goes into a state of total relaxation, which looks like sleep. Usually, a few minutes later, the patient can be roused to some extent, but it may be half an hour or more before full consciousness is restored. Once the patient has fully regained consciousness there may be a further phase during which he is somewhat confused, cannot quite remember what has happened, and complains of a headache.

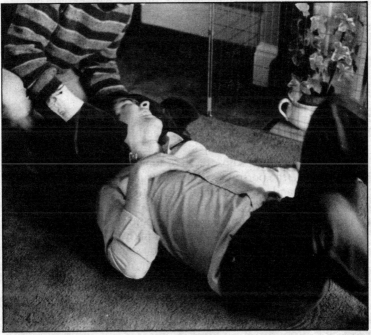

Fig 1 Patient's head being protected during a fit

How to help

What, therefore, should you do if you see someone have such a fit? Firstly you should remember that almost invariably the fit will not last long. The maximum duration is likely to be under five minutes, at the end of which the person will recover consciousness but may feel fairly drowsy and confused. It is most important that you should remain calm and keep those about you calm. Very often it is quite unnecessary to do anything but there are certain simple measures which can help considerably.

1 Ensure that the person having the fit is out of harm's way. Move him from the edge of a pavement or out of the way of electric wires or cables.
2 Cushion the head with something soft, such as a jacket, pillow or even your own arms.
3 Loosen any tight clothing round the neck, but do this gently rather than in a jerky manner.
4 Once the convulsions have ceased, turn the patient onto his side and place the head sideways too.
5 Somebody should stay with the person until he regains consciousness, when he should be helped into a chair so that he may relax until he feels able to carry on his business.

There are also some things you should not do.

1 Never try to restrain the jerking movements.
2 Never force anything between the teeth. This used to be done to prevent the person biting his tongue, but it is more likely to damage the patient's lips, teeth or tongue instead.
3 Do not give the person anything to drink during a fit. It will not help at all, and may even make the patient choke, vomit or swallow the fluid into his lungs.
4 Do not send for an ambulance or a doctor unless the fit does not end. If the whole episode is over in five minutes or so, you will usually find that, on regaining consciousness, the patient will be embarrassed about the incident, not wish to have any particular help, and soon continue on his way. However, if one fit succeeds another, the condition is potentially serious and you would be quite justified in sending for an ambulance. If necessary, dial 999, because such a patient will need expert hospital attention to bring him out of his successive fits.

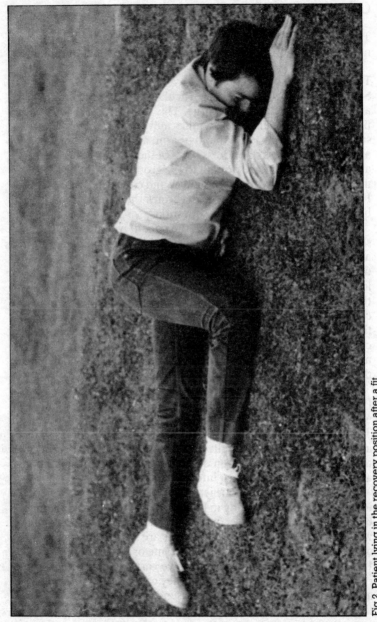

Fig 2 Patient lying in the recovery position after a fit

Other forms of epilepsy

There are other types of epileptic attacks when the whole body is not so affected, including two forms which are relatively common.

Temporal lobe epilepsy

Such an attack occurs when a particular portion of the brain is affected by an epileptic discharge. This sort of attack is shown by a patient having localised involuntary movements, such as lip smacking, twitching of the hand or arm, and odd movements, such as attempts to dress or undress parts of the body. A person may appear to be conscious, not fall to the ground and yet have the major type of fit, with severe rigidity and convulsive movements. However, during the course of the attack the patient is unlikely to be able to speak or respond to questions.

During a temporal lobe attack the patient will often feel a strange sensation, be in a rather dream-like state, and may at times act in a purposeful but totally meaningless manner. Very occasionally, people suffering from temporal lobe epilepsy may act in a violent or antisocial manner and retain no memory of this thereafter. I must emphasise that this is extremely rare, but of course such a pattern of behaviour is the one which is likely to hit the headlines in the local paper if and when it occurs. This can cause considerable unhappiness to all epilepsy sufferers who have never had, and know they never will have, an attack which affects them in this way.

Petit mal

Most people would not consider these attacks to be epileptic at all. The episode usually lasts for about 10 or 15 seconds and is so brief and undramatic that it usually passes unnoticed. Such *absences*, as they are usually called, often occur very frequently in childhood and generally do not persist into adult life.

They are caused by a transient loss of consciousness. For instance, the child working in his classroom just sits still looking blankly ahead for a few seconds and then carries on with what he was doing before. Because the attacks are so undramatic, it can well be that they are not noticed at home or at school. Unfortunately, such children can have very frequent attacks, and of course if this happens at school they can miss a significant amount of teaching because the absence is not noticed. As a result, they can be accused of being lazy, mischievous, inattentive or dim.

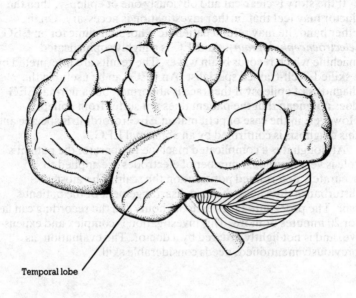

Temporal lobe

Fig 3 Diagram of brain showing the temporal lobe

Diagnosis

The diagnosis of epileptic attacks is made almost entirely on the case history. This, of course, will have to be given almost entirely by onlookers, so it is important when visiting the doctor that the patient is accompanied by a friend or relative who has witnessed these attacks. Quite often, attacks of loss of consciousness are not due to epilepsy, and can instead be due to a simple faint. It is only by going through the story in some detail that the doctor will be able to discover exactly how the whole situation has developed.

The physical examination of such patients invariably shows nothing of significance. The investigation of epileptic attacks depends upon age, and the particular type of attack. A febrile convulsion in a young child, for instance, often needs no investigation at all. The specific infection is treated and usually that is the end of the matter, with the parents often receiving advice about future prevention.

If the story is clear-cut and obviously one of epilepsy, then the doctor may feel that further investigation is necessary. On the other hand, he may refer a patient to a hospital clinic for an EEG (*electroencephalogram*). An EEG is a highly sophisticated machine which records brain waves. The results are interpreted by a skilled, well-trained specialist. An EEG can be useful in the diagnosis of epilepsy if the trace is abnormal, but a normal EEG does not mean that the patient does not suffer from epilepsy. However, in the case of petit mal an EEG recording is specific and this diagnosis is confirmed by an abnormal EEG.

Although it is a complicated machine to operate, the patient's role is very simple. A number of electrodes are applied to accurately determined positions on the scalp. The most disturbance this causes is some disarrangement of the patient's hair. The procedure takes up to an hour, and the recording can last for 20 minutes or more. This investigation is complex and expensive, and is not lightly ordered by a doctor. The evaluation, as previously mentioned, needs considerable skill.

Fig 4 Electrodes placed on patient's scalp for EEG reading

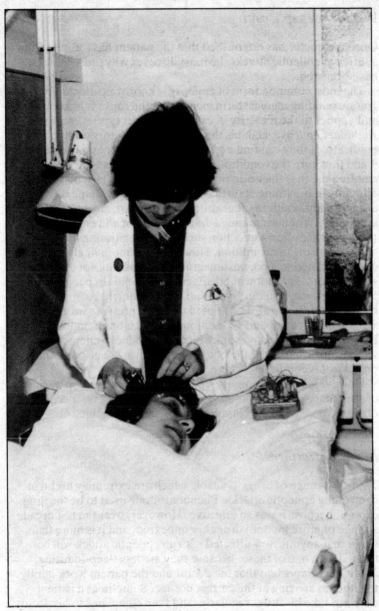

Neurophysiology Department, The Maudsley Hospital

What causes epilepsy?

Once the doctor has established that the patient has suffered from a series of epileptic attacks, he must discover why those attacks have occurred.

The most common form of epilepsy is known as *idiopathic*. This grand-sounding medical term means that the cause is unknown, and applies to the majority of cases. The other type is known as *secondary epilepsy*, and it is this form which doctors want to eradicate. If they can find a specific cause, then they can eliminate it and thus cure the condition. It is possible that in very young children the fit is due to an injury at birth, or to a lack of oxygen or difficulty in breathing at birth, as well as the high temperature already mentioned. In older children the fits are most likely to be idiopathic. When examining adults, the doctor will ensure that there is no significant infection such as meningitis or a brain abscess causing the condition. However, it is more likely that the cause is related to a preexisting injury, such as a motor cycle or car accident, or a gunshot wound affecting the head. In people over 50, epilepsy can also be a symptom of a haemorrhage or clot in a blood vessel. It can also be related to raised pressure inside the skull, which accompanies conditions such as a brain tumour. There is a range of chemical poisons which can produce epilepsy, and various disturbances of the body's metabolism are also known to produce this condition.

However, I must emphasise that although there are many causes of secondary epilepsy, in the vast majority of cases no specific cause is known and the condition is labelled idiopathic.

Medical treatment

There is a range of drugs available which are extremely useful in controlling epileptic attacks. Phenobarbitone used to be the drug chosen, because it was so effective. However, over the last decade a range of more modern drugs has appeared, and it is more than likely that anyone now affected with an epileptic attack will be treated with one of these, because they are less sleep-inducing.

It is very important that the doctor and the patient work jointly together in arriving at the correct dosage. Sometimes a patient does not take his drugs regularly, and then complains to his doctor that he is still suffering attacks. If the patient does not reveal the casualness of his drug taking, the doctor may increase the dosage in an attempt to control the condition. Such a pattern can obviously do the patient no good.

In the vast majority of cases, the attacks can be controlled by the careful selection of one drug, or a combination of drugs. Obviously this will not apply in all cases, and at times it is necessary for a patient to be admitted to hospital, where his progress can be monitored and his medication changed in controlled circumstances. In other cases, when the attacks are relatively infrequent, such as every three or four months, it can be deemed best not to place the patient on continuous medication, because it is so difficult to assess its effectiveness.

This illustrates that there is no one simple answer to the drug treatment of epilepsy, and that the competence of the doctor has to be complimented by the competence, interest and involvement of the patient and relatives.

Once the therapy has been started, it is essential that it is maintained regularly for between 18 months and two years after the last attack. Thereafter, with the doctor's consent, it is possible to reduce the drug dosage very slowly with a view to ceasing all medication over a period of another two years or so. This very gradual withdrawal of drugs is essential, because too fast a reduction of treatment could trigger off a further epileptic attack or series of attacks. Such attacks could well be unrelated to the original problem. In a very small percentage of cases, patients suffering from persistent severe epileptic attacks which do not respond to medication are candidates for specialised brain surgery.

Living with epilepsy

Although the drug therapy for epilepsy is often extremely effective, one of the major problems which affects sufferers and their doctors is convincing the family and friends, and especially the employer, that the patient is fit, safe, and well enough to lead an active and normal life. I think it is most important that the patient discusses his condition freely and openly with those around him. It is likely to cause him extreme embarrassment and potential difficulty if he has an attack and has not explained that this is likely to occur. It is far better for him to explain to his friends, colleagues and employer how an epileptic fit affects him, the likelihood of a fit occurring, how they should deal with one, and so on.

Employees and employers who have been warned are much more likely to be sympathetic, tolerant and helpful if an attack does occur.

If the facts are not explained, a patient might well find himself ostracized and criticized. There is always prejudice directed towards abnormality, and although it is totally untrue, people at times still think that others suffering from epilepsy are somewhat odd, mad or mentally defective. The fact that some very intelligent, fit, strong people have suffered from epilepsy has not helped to remove this unfortunate prejudice.

Leisure pursuits

In my opinion, a person who has had epileptic fits in the past, which are now properly treated, should be encouraged to lead as normal a life as possible. There is little point in having a condition well controlled and then being constantly told by parents and friends that one must not walk, run, climb, swim, sail or whatever. It is obvious that if a patient is going to take part in an activity which could be hazardous, someone should keep an eye on him, in case he has an unexpected attack.

Driving

With regard to driving, however, it is not a question of my personal opinion, because there are legal implications. Fortunately, the law has recently changed, and since 1974 licences have been granted to people with a history of epilepsy rather more easily than before. The history of epilepsy must be declared on the application form, and the patient must prove that:

1 He is free from epileptic attacks while awake.
2 He has had attacks only while asleep during the last three years.
3 If he drives a vehicle by himself, he will not endanger the public.

His own doctor will be asked to complete a form to substantiate his claims, and there are various other procedures which must be completed before the person can receive a driving licence.

I hope that throughout this chapter I have shown that epilepsy is a wide-ranging condition. The diagnosis is relatively easy and usually the treatment is very effective. The person so affected should be encouraged to lead as normal and active a life as possible, and his relatives, friends, employer, colleagues at work and the community at large should accept that he is likely to be as healthy and intelligent as everyone else. His only disability is epilepsy, which hopefully is now fully controlled.

I will finish with a quotation from the British Epilepsy Association. 'How many epileptics are there in Britain? None. But there are 300,000 people with epilepsy and some of them have fits. The fits are epileptic, not the people who have them.'

Varicose Veins

All of us have seen the unsightly bulging veins on other people's legs and probably wondered why they are there and why they have not been treated. This chapter deals with the causes of varicose veins, their prevention and treatment. Varicose veins are common, and many of us can expect to be troubled by them at some point in our lives. However, most of us do not need to suffer or fear the unsightly veins that I mentioned in the first sentence.

Before describing in detail what varicose veins are, I will first look at the normal circulation in the leg.

Blood circulation in the legs

The blood from the heart is pumped down into the legs along large arteries. It is the action of the heart which forces the blood onwards. The blood leaves the very small arteries and enters tiny blood vessels, known as *capillaries*, where the oxygen and chemicals in the blood diffuse out into muscle tissue. Now the blood begins to make its way back to the heart, and the pump action of the heart is no longer helpful. From the capillaries, the blood moves into small veins, and then into the larger ones which pass up the legs into the body cavity proper. Finally, it re-enters the heart.

The blood in the veins is forced upwards by the muscular action of walking. If one could observe the veins then, one would see that every time the muscles in the calf retract, the blood in the deep veins is forced upwards towards the heart. When the muscles relax, the blood from the outer veins is able to flow inward into the deep veins. Once in the deep veins, the blood is prevented from passing back to the outer surface of the leg by valves present in the communicating veins. These are the short veins which communicate between the outer and the inner venous systems. When these communicating valves fail, and the valves in the outer superficial veins fail, blood starts to accumulate and stagnate.

This is the beginning of varicose veins. Initially, there will be a slight bump or bulge, usually at the point where one of the communicating veins penetrates the leg muscles. Gradually, a length of superficial vein distends, and if the condition continues, lengths of vein stand out.

Why do these valves fail? There are various reasons, some of which are preventable and some of which are not.

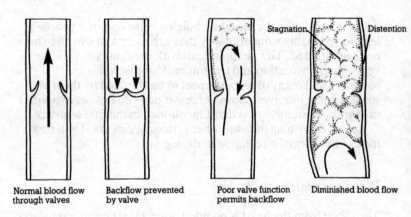

Normal blood flow through valves

Backflow prevented by valve

Poor valve function permits backflow

Diminished blood flow

Fig 5 Action of normal and failed valves in the leg

Potential sufferers

Heredity

Varicose veins can be hereditary. Some families are much more likely to suffer from varicose veins than others. If one's family does have a history of this condition, there is little one can do about it, except not aggravate the problem.

Prolonged standing

The most common cause of varicose veins is prolonged standing. If one remembers that the basic way of forcing blood up the veins is by walking, one will understand that if somebody has to stand for long periods, it will be difficult for the blood to pass up the legs. This means that the problem affects housewives who have to stand for long periods in the kitchen. In the past, policemen were also affected if they had to stand for long periods while on duty. I have noticed that now they rarely suffer because they either have desk jobs or patrol in cars.

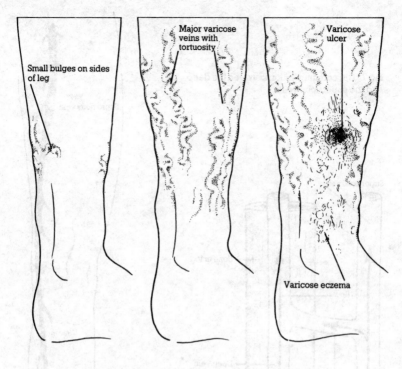

Fig 6 Legs showing the three stages of varicosity

Obesity

Anyone who is overweight is also a potential sufferer. He is likely to exercise less, to stand and rest more, and will also have more fatty tissue throughout the body. The obvious answer is to lose weight, but as those who are obese will know, this is easier said than done. I would like to say, however, that basically losing weight is a matter of eating less and exercising more, and I am certain that any doctor will be delighted to help with this problem.

Pregnancy

Pregnant women are also liable to develop varicose veins. There is no doubt that women who become pregnant two or three times will have some degree of varicosity in their legs. The reason is easily understood, because for the duration of the pregnancy, the return of blood from the legs to the body is somewhat impeded by the baby and the surrounding tissue in the lower abdomen.

27

Fig 7 The communication between the deep and the superficial veins

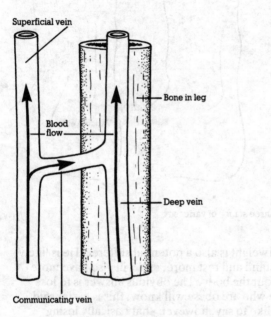

Superficial vein

Bone in leg

Blood flow

Deep vein

Communicating vein

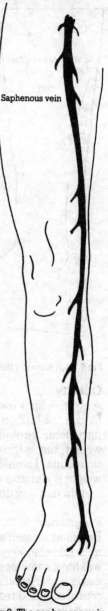

Saphenous vein

Fig 8 The saphenous vein

Constipation

In a similar way, it is thought that people suffering from chronic constipation are also prone to varicose veins. Certainly they are much more likely to suffer from piles (haemorrhoids), which are really the equivalent sort of bulging at the bottom of the large bowel in the region of the anus, but that is another story.

Diagnosis

There really is little problem in diagnosing the presence of varicose veins. They are either present or they are not. One merely has to look at the legs to determine the degree, nature and severity of the condition. I have seen quite a few young patients, particularly girls, who believe that they have varicose veins when in fact they have not. They think that because they can see the line of a vein under the skin, they have varicose veins. This is not so. In order to make a diagnosis, there must be a definite palpable bulge, which must be shown to be due to a defect in the filling of the vein.

Why then do patients come to the doctor with this condition? Often it is because a young mother is worried by the sight of small bulging varicosities in her legs. Although they do not give her any trouble, she has seen older women with much worse legs than hers and does not want her legs to become as bad. I think it is important to reassure her that as long as she takes reasonable exercise and does not have a whole host of children, it is unlikely that her varicose veins will steadily worsen and become too severe. One could also tactfully suggest that she keeps an eye on her weight over the years.

However, some people's veins do deteriorate and they suffer from other symptoms. The usual story is that there is a sense of persistent discomfort in the leg. The patient has a feeling of fatigue on walking and this can become generalized so that he no longer enjoys the activity as much as he once did. Because the veins are not working efficiently, the blood does not leave the legs as quickly as it should, and part of the blood, the *plasma*, can accumulate in the lower leg, particularly around the ankle. The patient will complain of swelling of the ankle and leg, and this adds to the discomfort. If the swelling persists, complications of varicose veins can develop.

29

Complications

Varicose eczema

Large untreated varicose veins can produce considerable swelling in the ankle area. As a result of the swelling, the skin can become thin and discoloured and what is known as varicose eczema can develop. This is a skin condition produced by the stagnant circulation and though the eczema can be helped with local preparations, the only effective cure is to deal with the varicose veins.

Varicose ulcers

If the skin thinning and stagnation persist for some years, the skin will break down and ulcerate. Varicose ulcers are unpleasant. They are difficult to deal with but respond very well to energetic treatment.

Haemorrhages

Varicose veins which have been present for some while, causing the skin to thin and bulge, can bleed. A minor knock to such a vein can produce a large and potentially frightening *haemorrhage*. The treatment is simple, consisting of making the patient lie down comfortably and lifting the leg into the air. Pressure is then applied to the area which is bleeding, using a clean handkerchief or other suitable clean dressing material. The bleeding will stop almost immediately.

This is obvious if one thinks about it because, as already explained, the blood circulation in the vein depends on muscle movement. If one elevates the limb and presses on the bleeding area to stop the movement, the blood circulation in that area will stop at once. A firm bandage is then applied to the area. The patient should then consult his doctor for more definite treatment of the whole condition.

Clotting

More serious is the problem of clotting, or *thrombosis*, in the veins. The dangers of this condition have been widely discussed over the past few years. Fortunately, this is not a common problem and when it does happen it develops slowly and almost always responds to medical treatment. The symptoms are that a particular segment of the vein becomes hard and tender. On examination, this firm tender area feels rather like a pencil, in comparison to the rest of the veins which are soft and not tender. The immediate treatment of such a condition, known as *phlebitis*, is to rest the leg, which of course also means resting the patient. If the affected veins are not directly connected to the main body system, the chances are very favourable for a quick recovery.

However, the risk is that the clotting, or thrombosis, can extend from a superficial vein into a deep vein. This is a much more serious problem and the whole question of deep vein thrombosis is beyond the scope of this chapter. Suffice to say it is a serious condition which almost certainly warrants hospital admission and the use of drugs to reduce the tendency of the blood to clot.

Minor treatment of varicose veins

There is a tremendous variety of treatments available for varicose veins, ranging from the very simple to the complicated. I will start with the easiest and work through to the hardest.

Exercise

If a person visits me with minimal varicose veins, which cause little or no trouble at all, I suggest that the best thing is to forget all about them and continue living normally as before. There is no need to embark on specific treatments and one hopes that the condition will not worsen. One can suggest that the patient might take more exercise and lose any excess weight, but that is really all one needs to do for a mild case of varicose veins.

If the condition is somewhat more troublesome, there is a variety of options open.

Support stockings and bandages

One can suggest that the patient wears a supporting stocking or bandage during the day, which often gives all the support necessary. For instance, if the patient combines this support with more vigorous exercise and weight reduction, if necessary, the problem can be reduced significantly, although of course the vein will never completely vanish.

Stockings and bandages are obtainable from one's general practitioner under the National Health Service, and most chemists stock a range, or can order them. Obviously such stockings and bandages must be looked after with care, and the manufacturer's instructions should be read carefully. In order to obtain the maximum help from such supportive measures, the bandage or stockings must be put on first thing in the morning when the leg is not swollen. If they need to be reapplied or changed during the day, the leg should be elevated for half an hour or so first.

Vein injections

The simplest medical treatment consists of injecting the veins, if the problem areas are not too large and too many. The technique consists of the surgical specialist defining the exact positions of the varicose areas, injecting the venous bulge and then applying a pressure bandage. The patient is asked to take a vigorous daily walk for up to 3 miles (5km) and the firm compression bandage is left on the leg for at least a week. The vein is then reinspected by the surgeon, who may decide to reinject the same area before injecting the other veins. The particular pattern of injection and solution used varies according to the surgeon, as does the degree of exercise and compression prescribed, and length of time during which the patient is under observation.

The injection techniques generally work well, and the patient needs to clearly follow the advice given. At the same time, it has to be accepted that although this treatment has a very good track record, it does not give an absolute guarantee of cure and the patient can develop more varicose veins years later.

Hospital treatment

If the surgeon considers that the injection techniques are not going to be adequate, he will suggest hospital admission in order to follow a more elaborate procedure. This can vary in complexity.

Tying the vein

The simplest treatment consists of tying the superficial vein in the upper thigh, thereby preventing the flow of blood in the superficial vein, and deflecting it into the deeper veins.

Stripping the vein

However, the simple blocking of part of one long vein is usually not sufficient, and this basically simple operation has been developed over the years so that now, as well as the incision and tying up of the vein, one also advocates what is known as stripping the vein. This consists of the removal of the long vein.

During the operation an instrument known as a stripper is passed up or down the long superficial vein. When this has been carefully done, the instrument is removed, stripping out the vein at the same time. Very firm pressure has to be applied to the leg thereafter, and the patient will obviously have to accept some degree of discomfort in the leg for two or three days after the operation.

After the operation, the bottom of the patient's bed is raised by about 10°. The patient is encouraged to walk around on the first day, wearing a bulky pressure bandage. Thereafter, this is likely to be replaced by a firm elastic bandage, which is applied directly to the leg. The patient stays in hospital, depending upon the amount of discomfort in the leg, the home circumstances and the surgeon's own particular preferences, for between two and seven days.

Very often the patient is able to return home still wearing the bandages and dressings. Later, under the supervision of the general practitioner and district nurse, the stitches can be removed at home quite easily. Following this convalescent period, the patient is encouraged to walk regularly, not to stand for long, and to rest at regular intervals with the leg elevated. It is likely that the patient will be advised to wear firm supportive bandages around the leg for at least four weeks.

Therefore, what appears to be a relatively simple condition is dealt with by a variety of techniques, the most serious being the complete removal of the affected vein.

Operations on varicose veins are no longer regarded as relatively unimportant and there are now many skilled surgeons who devote a considerable amount of their time to dealing with this problem.

Treatment of varicose ulcers

The treatment of varicose ulcers is bound to be difficult because they only arise when the condition has been present for some time. The doctor will almost certainly wish to reduce the patient's weight, and encourage exercise as well as treat the ulcer. Once the ulcer is clean, with the appropriate dressings applied, the surgeon will decide whether to treat the varicose veins and the ulcer together, or tackle the varicose veins first and see if the ulcer will heal on its own as a result. It is possible to apply skin grafts to varicose ulcers, but such grafting is highly unlikely to be successful if the problem of severe varicose veins persists. However, this is a complex problem and is best treated by a surgical team both interested and skilled in dealing with this condition.

The basic message then is that although varicose veins are something that many people can expect to have, they should not cause too much trouble. They can be prevented from becoming too severe if one avoids standing for long periods, takes a reasonable amount of exercise, and keeps a close watch on one's weight. If one is troubled with them, it is far better to consult one's doctor early, rather than to wait until one's legs are painful, swollen and discoloured. One should always be seen by a doctor long before a varicose ulcer develops. If enough preventative steps are taken, such ulcers will become things of the past over the next few years.

Constipation

The British are obsessed with constipation. I do not know how
many different laxatives and purgatives are sold in this country per
year, but it is certainly a vast quantity, and mostly quite
unnecessary. Many people feel that it is essential to go to the toilet
at least once a day in order to live a healthy life. There is a
widespread belief that if the bowels do not open in this way, one
will become poisoned and suffer terrible illnesses. If the time and
energy expended in thinking about our bowels was channelled into
something more constructive, we would all be a lot happier. Of
course it is necessary to pass faeces but there is no definite rule
which states exactly how often one should do so. It depends
entirely on how much one eats, what one eats and what sort of
bowel opening habit one has developed over the years.

What is constipation?

I think it might be defined as a delay in the evacuation of the large
bowel, shown by the production of hard, dryish faeces. Is this
necessarily bad? The answer must be no, unless the pattern is
persistently maintained. At times we all may find that for two or
three days we do not go to the toilet and then when we do we pass
a hard firm motion which may give some pain. This is not harmful,
unless one is chronically constipated, when a variety of problems
can develop.

Fuel for the body

In order to live we must eat. We eat to absorb enough energy
replacement in the form of carbohydrates and fats, and to take in
specific proteins, in the form of amino acids, which will help to
build up our bodies and to replace tissue which is constantly being
worn out. A growing child or young adolescent needs considerably
more food than an adult because, as well as repairing the daily

wear and tear, he has a tremendous need for protein to build and
develop his body as it steadily gets bigger and stronger. At the
same time, because he is so active, his energy requirements are
great and consequently he needs food containing carbohydrates.

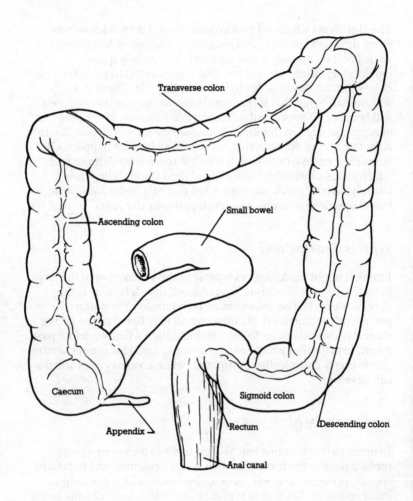

Fig 9 The colon, rectum and anus

The digestion process

Food is crushed and chewed in the mouth until it is small enough to be swallowed, when it passes into the stomach. Once it has been broken down into smaller units, it passes on into the small intestine. As it makes its way through this long tortuous tube, more of the chemical goodness is absorbed, so that by the time the residue reaches the large bowel the food is *denatured* and one is left with the waste products. This passage through the small intestine, which is about 20ft (6m) long, takes a variable time, depending upon the type of food and the activity of the person in question. The residue then passes into the colon, or the large bowel, which is about 5ft (1.5m) of large intestine, 2½″ (6cm) wide.

If the diet has been wholesome, and not the highly refined food which so many people tend to eat these days, there will be a considerable bulk of residue passing up into the colon. This mass is large, soft, and full of fluid. The muscles in the colon wall are able to contract on the bulky matter and can force it steadily up the ascending colon, along the transverse colon, and down the descending colon into the rectum.

When a sufficient amount of bulky mass is present in the rectum, a nervous reflex is initiated which signals a desire to go to the toilet to the conscious mind. If one heeds this desire then one is able to pass the contents of the rectum easily.

However, because of the hustle and bustle of daily life and because often one is not prepared to allow sufficient time for an important natural activity, one does not bother to go to the toilet when one receives the reflex urge. As a result, the faeces tend to accumulate in the rectum. The longer they stay there, the greater the quantity, and potentially the more difficult they are to pass. This is because the fluid in the bulky mass begins to be reabsorbed into the body. Eventually one produces the hard, rather dry faecal mass which is characteristic of constipation.

Causes of constipation

I have already mentioned one significant cause, which is the failure to respond to the reflex. The reflex is normally stimulated by a large meal, when it is known as the *gastro-colic reflex*. When we eat well and fill our stomachs, this produces a reflex contraction of the large bowel, resulting in the desire to go to the toilet. You will surely have noticed that between 20 minutes and half an hour after a meal, you often wish to go to the toilet. If you are in a crowded hotel or restaurant, you may well find that many others feel the same way and suddenly you are in trouble because all the lavatories are occupied.

Diet

What else causes constipation? The other most common cause, and probably the most important, is the faulty diet which most of us tend to have in this country. We are the victims of our own success. At about the beginning of this century millers were able to produce white flour through a process of refining, removing the husk from the wheat grain. Our grandparents no longer had to eat coarse bread, given the choice of gleaming white loaves. This fashion has continued so that now most of us have been conditioned to eat this bread, which I find can be spongy and tasteless. However, although I dislike the taste of it and do my best to avoid it, my children thoroughly disagree with me.

Be that as it may, whether you like or dislike the taste of white bread, the fact remains that it has been purified, lacks fibre, and therefore lacks bulk. Although it is rich in carbohydrate and often has added vitamins, making it a valuable food, white bread is of little or no value to the large bowel. Our bodies were designed thousands of years ago, and have not yet caught up with today's plasticised, supermarket age. The bowel needs a bulky diet in order to act comfortably. If this is not present, the bowel becomes sluggish, is unable to produce adequate reflexes, and will cause constipation.

The truth of this argument is well illustrated by comparing the bowel actions of Western Europeans with those of Africans living in rural parts of Africa. Whatever disadvantages they may suffer, and there are many, one of them is certainly not constipation. Their diet is rough and coarse, and they tend to have large soft motions on a regular basis every day. Whereas the civilised person living in Western Europe may only pass 2oz (50g) of faeces a day, a rural African can pass well over 1lb (450g) of faeces at one time.

What is probably of greater interest is the time taken for the food to pass through the alimentary system from mouth to anus. It has been shown that the passage of food from mouth to anus takes about 24 hours in a rural African, whereas it takes up to three days in Western Europeans. Linked almost certainly with this is the fact that Western Europeans suffer from diseases of the large and small bowel such as *appendicitis, diverticulitis* and cancer of the colon, which are all virtually unheard of in rural African villages. While I am not suggesting that one should live in an African village, I do think we would all improve our health considerably if we ate a more natural diet. I will come back to this again later.

Other causes

Other causes of constipation are not as common, but are facts which should be known and noted.

Pregnancy

Pregnant women tend to have difficulties with their bowels, which is not surprising when one considers that the developing baby presses on the colon, and to some degree obstructs the passage of motions within it. It is best dealt with by ensuring that the diet is bulky, that the expectant mother has plenty of fruit, vegetables and fluids, and leads as active a life as possible.

Emotional causes

A change of environment can cause either diarrhoea or constipation, depending upon one's personality, how one eats and what one drinks. One of the common symptoms of a depressive illness is constipation. However, this is usually such a minor part of the whole illness that it is almost unremarked upon by the patient.

Drugs

Unfortunately, some drugs produce constipation as a side effect. If a patient who previously has had no such problems is placed on drugs and thereafter becomes constipated, he should discuss the matter with his doctor. One of the common medicines producing this side effect is iron, given for iron deficiency anaemia.

Obsession

Another cause of constipation is the obsessional preoccupation with the condition which affects some people. They become so interested in their bowel actions that unwittingly they produce the very condition they are trying to avoid.

Old age

As one grows older, one tends to eat and drink less, and one's bowel muscles become weaker. Therefore, in old age particularly, if one is not feeling well, constipation can intrude and make life more unpleasant.

Examination

Constipation has a variety of causes and can be a problem for a short or long time. I think that a person who feels that he is constipated, and has been so for more than one or two weeks, should consult his doctor. Very often, the doctor will be able to reassure him that he is not constipated at all. This can easily be done, by placing one hand on the abdomen to detect whether the large bowel is full of faeces or not, followed by an examination of the back passage to see if this is loaded with hard or soft faeces. If the diagnosis of constipation has been made, the condition must be treated.

Treatment

Mild laxatives
If the patient has not been taking laxatives on a regular basis, this is an occasion when a simple laxative could be effective. I would suggest to such a patient that he took two tablets in the evening, with plenty to drink, in order to give the bowel some extra fluid. By next morning, a firm bowel action should have been passed and the problem solved.

Stronger laxatives and suppositories
However, if the patient habitually takes laxatives, the use of simple laxatives is unlikely to be effective when he does become genuinely constipated. A more powerful laxative would be prescribed, again taken with plenty of fluids. If this failed, one would prescribe a suppository which could be inserted into the back passage once or twice.

Enema
If neither of these methods worked, the doctor might have to arrange for a district nurse to give the patient an enema. This can be done quite simply today, often using a prepared pack of fluid which is squeezed into the back passage through a tube and

40

retained there. The action of the fluid with the drug therapy which it contains will produce a good bowel action within a relatively short time.

Manual evacuation

Very occasionally the constipation is so intractable and the motion so hard that the only way to deal with the situation is by manual evacuation. This is the insertion of the fingers into the back passage, and the breaking up and removal of the motion piecemeal. This can usually be done quite simply, but very occasionally such a patient has to be admitted to hospital for the procedure. Thereafter, the whole question of diet in relation to constipation is explained in detail to the patient.

Preventing constipation

I think it is obvious that I have strong views on this subject. It seems to me that although constipation is a common problem, it can easily be prevented. It is not unreasonable to suggest that instead of eating white processed bread one should eat wholemeal bread instead. The use of fresh fruit and vegetables gives added roughage to one's diet. It is far better to eat fresh foods which have the extra roughage, than to eat the anaemic canned variety which is prepared to look attractive but from which all extra fibre has been removed. If these simple measures do not produce adequate bowel actions, one should add bran to one's diet.

Bran in the diet

Bran is the outer coating of the wheat grain and is, as mentioned previously, removed in the production of white bread. It is a source of cereal fibre and it produces the added bulk which can help to prevent constipation. It can be purchased from chemists, grocers and supermarkets.

One starts cautiously by adding one or two teaspoonsful of it a day to water, milk or cereals. It can even be included in casseroles and stews. It is advisable not to begin with too large a dose because this can produce too much bulk and cause colic pains. It is also necessary to drink at least an extra pint (½ litre) of liquid a day so that the bran can be absorbed in this to produce the necessary

41

bulk. The actual amount of bran that one needs is only found by trial and error, but the more roughage one takes in one's ordinary diet the less bran one needs. There is no doubt that this is a safe, simple, natural and effective way of keeping the bowels open and it is also cheap. Bran can be obtained generally throughout the country.

Constipation as a symptom

In conclusion, I think I should comment on constipation from the doctor's point of view. In the main, as I have mentioned often in this chapter, it is a preventable problem. However, as far as I am concerned, any patient who comes to see me with a significant alteration of bowel habit must be examined carefully in order to ensure there is not any serious underlying condition. If somebody whose bowel habits have previously been perfectly regular develops a pattern of constipation, or constipation alternating with diarrhoea, then a visit to the doctor is necessary in order to ensure the problem is not being caused by a physical blockage or obstruction in part of the large bowel. If in doubt, therefore, I would suggest making an appointment with one's doctor. The problem could well be simple and solved easily, thereafter making one's life much happier for years. On the other hand, if there is anything significant developing, the sooner it is seen, assessed and treated, the better.

Improving Your Diet

Instead of viewing this chart as a temporary measure, make it your new long-term eating plan. All the foods suggested on these pages are healthy, full of essential vitamins and other nutrients, good sources of fibre, and most of them are relatively cheap. They are also very bulky, so you will find that less food is more satisfying.

Essential foods

Fresh fruit and vegetables play a large part in this diet, but they must be prepared properly. Eat them raw whenever possible, and preferably unskinned. Most of the goodness lies just under the skin, which is also an excellent source of fibre in itself. Vegetables should be cooked in as little water, and for as short a time, as

possible, in order to preserve their flavour and nutrients.
Your daily intake should include all of the following:
Breakfast cereals high in roughage
Wholemeal bread
Fresh fruit
Fresh vegetables
Plenty of fluids

Supplementary foods

Increase your intake of bran, initially starting with a teaspoonful at
a time, and increasing gradually by adding lose bran to stewed fruit
or soups. Experiment with the different varieties of pulses, but eat
them instead of meat at a meal.
Supplement your daily intake with some of the following:
Dried fruits (prunes, sultanas, apricots etc)
Nuts
Loose bran
Fruit juices
Pulses (beans, peas, lentils etc)
Brown rice

Foods and drinks to avoid

Make room for all these high-fibre foods by reducing your intake
of sweet foods. You may even find that you lose a little weight on
this new eating plan of high-fibre, healthy foods.
You should cut down on, or exclude completely, the following
foods:
Starchy puddings
Sweetened drinks
Sugar-based foods (biscuits, chocolate etc)
Crisps
Cakes

Bronchitis

As I began to write this chapter I had to stop because I was coughing. This irritated and annoyed me because I do not normally expect to cough but at least I know, or hope I know, that in two or three days the coughing will have stopped and I shall be reasonably fit again.

Why is this so? The answer is simple. I do not smoke. I am afraid that throughout this chapter the question of smoking will be mentioned and my dislike of it will be very apparent. It is not that I dislike the smell, because fortunately or not, I have a very poor sense of smell. The reason is far simpler. I intensely dislike seeing people deliberately destroying their own lungs when I know how difficult it will be for me to help them when eventually they become so breathless that no treatment will be of any value to them.

Smoking, particularly of cigarettes, is the basic cause of the most common form of cancer. Lung cancer kills far more people in one year in Great Britain than any other form of cancer. The tragedy is that it is almost certainly a form of cancer which, to a large extent, can be completely prevented.

However, I feel I have said enough about my views on smoking and cancer and in this chapter will not be developing the theme to any great extent. Instead, I will examine the question of lung diseases which are referred to under the name *bronchitis*.

What is bronchitis?

When I first started in general practice my patients were invariably frightened if I said they had bronchitis, but were far less troubled if I referred to their coughing and spluttering as being due to bronchial catarrh. Basically what is meant by bronchitis is an inflammation of the bronchial tubes.

Respiratory tract infections

The most common way in which inflammation and infection

45

affects the bronchial tubes in the lung, and lung tissue itself, is by the spread of infection from the mouth and throat. This area, together with the nasal air passages, is known as the upper respiratory tract. One of the problems that general practitioners have to deal with most often is the constant succession of patients troubled with *upper respiratory tract infections* (URTI).

Most of these infections are self limiting. That is a piece of medical jargon which really means that whatever you do, or do not do, you will recover in a few days. Everyone, particularly in the winter, can expect to suffer a few times from a stuffy nose, sore throat, general aches and pains, and this can quite often develop into a cough.

The cough is sometimes dry and harsh and can become moist, when *sputum* is coughed up from the lungs. The change from just the stuffy nose and sore throat to the development of a cough with the production of sputum signifies the change from an upper respiratory tract infection to one involving the lower respiratory tract; in order words, the lungs.

If a heavy infection develops, due to either bacteria or viruses, and the defensive tissues in the upper respiratory tract are unable to combat the infection, the whole tract is likely to become involved, and a cough will develop. It is also far more likely for this to develop if one is not particularly fit at the time. This can happen if one is overworked and somewhat run down, or if the lungs are basically not as strong as they might be due to continued damage from smoking, or to an inherent defect, such as asthma.

Treatment

The treatment of a respiratory tract disorder, which is a modern and somewhat long-winded term for an attack of acute bronchitis, is to rest, keep warm, drink plenty of liquids (excluding alcohol), take aspirin or paracetamol as necessary and to seek medical advice if the sputum is thick, and yellow or green.

The doctor hearing such a story will almost certainly prescribe the appropriate antibiotics, and will expect them to be taken on a regular basis for about a week. It is not possible to say that one particular antibiotic should be prescribed because bacteria vary in their sensitivity, and different parts of the country tend to be affected by varieties of bacteria in the same way that there are many regional dialects.

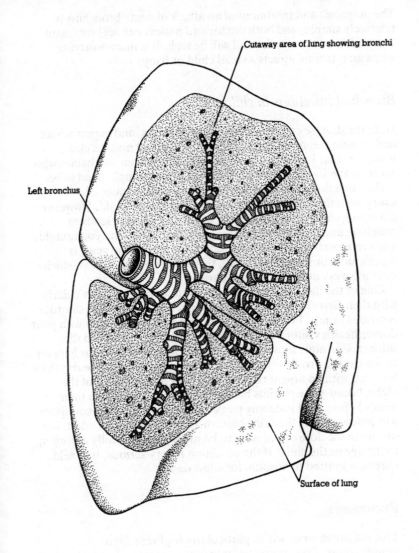

Cutaway area of lung showing bronchi

Left bronchus

Surface of lung

Fig 10 The bronchial tree of the left lung

47

The diagnosis and treatment of an attack of acute bronchitis is relatively simple, and both doctor and patient can feel confident that within a very few days all will be well. It is more worrying when an infection affects a small child or baby.

Bronchial infections in children

Here the disease can create significant distress, and expert advice and prompt treatment must be sought. I should make it clear, however, that I am not suggesting that all children and babies who produce the signs of a cold in the head, plus a cough, need to be rushed to a doctor. It is quite unnecessary and a waste of everyone's time, as well as being upsetting to the child. However, if a young child or baby develops a cold, which then leads to coughing and distress in breathing, it is likely that the young child, and more particularly the baby under the age of one year, is significantly unwell. Potentially, this is a serious condition which warrants very active treatment early.

One of the basic problems which troubles parents, particularly with their first child, is to decide when a respiratory tract disorder is serious or not. I think this is something you can discuss with your doctor/health visitor before it happens to get his views on the subject. Certainly most general practitioners would be far happier to discuss the problem with an anxious mother during the day than be faced with an urgent request for a visit in the middle of the night, because the parents had not been able to make up their minds before, and suddenly panic. Treatment of such a youngster will follow exactly the same pattern as described for an adult, but of course the dosage will have to be monitored carefully according to the age of the child. If the condition is very serious, the child may be admitted to hospital for a few days.

Pneumonia

This is a dread word which particularly frightened our grandparents. Prior to the last war patients affected with this disease were likely to die, unless they were basically very fit, because antibiotics were not yet available. Pneumonia is an infection, not of the bronchial tubes, but of the fine lung tissue (the alveoli or the air sacs). Pneumonia can be present either in

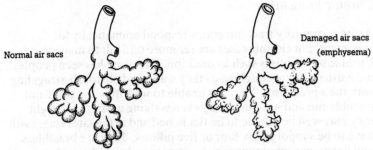

Normal air sacs

Damaged air sacs (emphysema)

Fig 11 Difference between normal and emphysematous air sacs

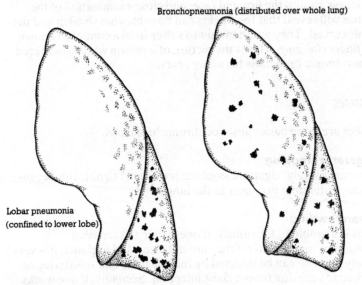

Bronchopneumonia (distributed over whole lung)

Lobar pneumonia (confined to lower lobe)

Fig 12 Areas affected by lobar and bronchopneumonia

scattered areas through the lung, when it is known as *broncho-pneumonia*, or confined to a more specific area, in which case it is known as *lobar pneumonia*.

A patient with pneumonia is usually more ill than one with acute bronchitis, and on examination of the lungs the doctor will be able to detect a patch of pneumonia by listening for any abnormal breath sounds. The treatment with modern antibiotics is usually extremely successful and the thought of pneumonia should no longer create the despondency it once did.

49

Chronic bronchitis

Acute respiratory tract infections respond dramatically to
treatment, but chronic cases are far more difficult to manage.
Chronic bronchitis is such a condition. Everyone has seen people,
most usually men, coughing as they walk, and obviously struggling
with their breathing. They are unable to walk quickly, could not
possibly run and have difficulty even walking upstairs. At night
they may well be unable to lie flat in bed and in the later stages will
have to be supported by four or five pillows. They are breathless
and have a chronic cough which varies from being dry and
unproductive to being moist and productive. Sometimes there is
blueness around the lips and face, and close examination of the
hands will reveal that the fingers can be somewhat swollen and the
nails curved. They are then said to suffer from a condition known
as *finger clubbing*. This is the picture of a person who has suffered
from chronic bronchitis for many years.

Causes

There are three basic causes of chronic bronchitis.

Cigarette smoking
Not surprisingly, cigarette smoking is the most significant, because
of the irritation it produces in the lungs.

Overcrowding
This is a problem. Obviously, if one is living in crowded
conditions, particularly if they are not clean and hygienic, it is very
likely that one can be infected by the coughing and spluttering of
someone suffering from a chest infection. Secondly, if one works
in a constantly dusty atmosphere, the lungs become chronically,
although mildly, irritated. The long-term effect produces some
degree of lung damage and some inflammation, and gives a likely
base to which infection can add trouble.

Air pollution
Working in and around big cities used to cause significant
problems because of the smoke, particularly the sulphur dioxide in
the air. Fortunately, this has been reduced significantly by govern-
ment acts over the last few years which have reintroduced clean air

to the large urban areas. I can remember vividly living in Birmingham, when the winter heralded evenings of such thick fog that it was impossible to move from my home to the surgery unless I walked. My main concern, however, was for my patients, who would get acute flare-ups of their bronchitis because the filth in the fog had reactivated it. Now, this is a thing of the past.

It is not my intention in this chapter to deal with industrial chest diseases, but I would just like to mention the problems which still face people such as coal miners, who have to work in dust-laden atmospheres, although the hazard to them has been significantly reduced over the past few years.

Typically, then, the chronic bronchitic patient is a man who has worked in a dusty atmosphere and who almost inevitably has been a heavy smoker for 10 years or more. The combination of the atmospheric and personal pollution has damaged his bronchial tree and the resultant inflammation has reduced his vital lung capacity. He is unable to breathe in and out as much air at one time as he once could. This means that when he is at rest, or doing moderate exercise, there is no problem. However, once he has to exercise more vigorously he finds that he becomes *hypoxic*. In other words, he is unable to get into his lungs as much oxygen as he needs to carry in his blood for vital purposes, and therefore puffs and blows and may well find that he has come to a standstill.

The result of the chronic inflammation of the bronchial tubes is that they secrete a mucous material, which is constantly coughed up as a clear, colourless fluid. When this becomes infected at intervals during the year, as it inevitably does, the colour changes from the previous clear mucous to a thin or thick yellow or green colour. If the patient normally works in a dust-laden atmosphere, the sputum can be always somewhat cloudy and never absolutely clear.

Emphysema

The constant pattern of inflammation, coughing and breathlessness damages the many small air sacs within the lung, and a condition known as *emphysema* develops. Such an emphysematous lung has fewer air sacs than normal, giving less available area within the lung for oxygen to diffuse from the air sacs into the capillaries.

51

This is what breathing is all about. If one cannot obtain an adequate supply of oxygen into one's body, and at the same time get rid of an equivalent amount of carbon dioxide, one has to reduce one's activities significantly. At the same time, when the damage increases beyond a certain point, it is likely that one's lips, tongue and possibly the face become bluish. If such a chronic state develops, life becomes increasingly unpleasant, one's energy drive is reduced, and one can lose weight.

Diagnosing chronic bronchitis

Therefore, the diagnosis of this condition is relatively easy. Almost inevitably, at some point, the general practitioner will arrange for a chest x-ray in order to ensure that the patient is not suffering from any more serious disorder. Once it has been established that he is not, there is little need to repeat the chest x-rays unless the doctor feels that there has been some significant change.

Treatment

Having established the diagnosis of chronic bronchitis, what advice can the doctor offer the patient? Firstly, one would deal with the immediate acute infection using an appropriate antibiotic. Secondly, one would try, and usually fail, to convince the patient that if his lungs are to improve or at least not to deteriorate, he must personally deal with the situation. He must stop smoking. He must avoid air pollution. This, of course, is very difficult if he is unable to move away from a dusty work atmosphere or if he lives in an area which still suffers from air pollution. However, if he is willing to give up smoking, I am sure that his doctor, friends and employers will be prepared to help him.

Vaccination

Obviously such people are at risk from recurrent chest infections in the winter, but they can be protected with influenza vaccines. If the breathing is significantly affected, some advice about breathing exercises may be helpful, but to expect physiotherapy as such to deal with the problem is obviously foolish.

Reducing weight

I have not mentioned a further factor which obviously will affect breathlessness, although it is not a cause of bronchitis, and that is obesity. Anybody who is suffering from difficulty in breathing can, of course, improve his general fitness by reducing his weight. If the patient combines this with a pattern of regular but reasonable exercise, he can maximise his fitness and keep himself in a reasonable condition.

I am afraid this is a gloomy chapter, but in spite of this I must finish by pointing out that unfortunately in severe cases of chronic bronchitis there is only a 30% expectation of survival within a five-year period. I hope by now I have convinced you to stop smoking, or if you are a non-smoker convinced you to convert the smokers in your family into non-smokers. This is vital in the prevention, and treatment, of chronic bronchitis. I think that smoking is a form of addiction and that one becomes dependent upon a raised blood nicotine level. It is, of course, far better never to have started and I think that parents should make quite certain that they do their very best to stop their children smoking and to set them an example.

However, if you are a smoker you can be helped by the various campaigns and anti-smoking clinics operated by many Area Health Authorities. I would suggest that you ask your doctor or contact your Area Health Authority direct.

Action on Smoking and Health (ASH) is an organisation which is very concerned about the prevention of smoking, and you can write direct to them for specific information. Finally, can I remind you that no matter how long you have smoked, it is always worthwhile giving it up. You will undoubtedly derive some benefit although obviously your lungs will never return to their previous level of perfection.

On the following pages is a chart of suggested ways of giving up smoking.

Giving Up Smoking

The best way to give up smoking is to just stop. Although it may sound impossible, it is really better than to cut down gradually, when you may find yourself tempted to have 'just one more' cigarette each day. The suggestions on these pages can apply to either method of stopping smoking, but do not include the vital element – willpower.

Work out how much money you would have spent in a year on cigarettes – it may now pay for your holiday

Each week, put the money you would have spent on cigarettes into a special jar, or building society account

Read about the damage cigarettes do to lungs

Give up smoking with a friend. You can then spur each other on

Do not make a fuss about giving up smoking. If anyone offers you a cigarette, thank them but say 'not at the moment'

Develop new hobbies to keep your mind alert and off cigarettes

Become more active so that you become fitter and won't want to ruin that by smoking again

Change your routine so that you won't miss cigarettes so much (drink tea instead of coffee, eat at a different time of the day etc)

Temporarily avoid socialising with friends who smoke

Travel in non-smoking sections on public transport

Sit in the non-smoking sections of cinemas and restaurants

Drink plenty of fresh orange juice. The vitamin C will help rid the body of nicotine

Eat fresh fruit or raw vegetables whenever you want a cigarette. This is less fattening and healthier than eating sweets

If you have to do something with your fingers, play with a ring, pencil, rubber band etc

If you really crave a cigarette, do deep breathing exercises until the urge passes.

Finally, if you feel you need outside support, you may wish to seek the potential help of hypnotherapy or the collective help of an organisation such as Action on Smoking and Health (ASH)

Multiple Sclerosis

Multiple sclerosis (also called *disseminated sclerosis*) is the most common disease affecting the nervous pathways in the brain and spinal cord. About 50,000 people are so affected in Great Britain. It is a disease which appears in many forms, and varies in its pattern of behaviour once it has developed.

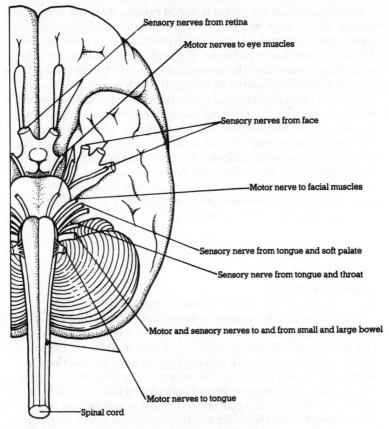

Sensory nerves from retina

Motor nerves to eye muscles

Sensory nerves from face

Motor nerve to facial muscles

Sensory nerve from tongue and soft palate

Sensory nerve from tongue and throat

Motor and sensory nerves to and from small and large bowel

Motor nerves to tongue

Spinal cord

Fig 13 Brain and spinal cord showing main nerve pathways

Any disease which manifests itself in many ways and has a very changeable course over the years presents significant problems to doctors, patients and relatives. This is particularly so when the variation is so great that at one end of the range is a patient who has one or two minimal attacks and then no more trouble for many years, and at the other a patient who unfortunately has severe recurrent attacks leading to significant disability in a relatively short time.

What causes multiple sclerosis?

The other significant problem is that at present the cause is not known. There are many theories and every two or three years some enthusiast produces another. Unfortunately, at present no definitive cause has been found, although I think there is probably general agreement that the disease is the result of some form of excessive tissue reaction to an infection which occured within the body some time, perhaps years, before the onset of the symptoms. However, even this sort of suggestion is very vague. The result is that no specific advice can be offered to people who wish to set up preventive programmes. At the same time, because no one knows the specific cause of the disease, the field is open to all sorts of misguided, and at times disreputable, people who produce their own theories with total confidence. Also, they invariably offer their own form of treatment and cure, usually at a significant cost to the unfortunate patient or relatives.

Physical symptoms

Visual disturbance
One of the most common symptoms is a visual disturbance. Typically, the disease appears in young adults, with the patient experiencing some visual difficulty in one eye associated with pain and discomfort. On examination, it is found that the patient has significant blurring or even loss of vision of one eye, and that the pain is specifically felt on the movement of the eyeball. As well as the general visual blurring, an optician testing the visual field of a patient will find that the central area of vision may be lost. The visual disturbance stops after about two or three weeks, although on subsequent testing a partial loss of central vision may be found

to persist. Later, when the back of the eye is examined once more with the ophthalmoscope, it can be found that there is a whitening of part of the optic disc. This abnormal process within the nervous system is caused by damage to the myelin sheaths which surround the nerves. The sheaths become swollen, damaged and scarred.

It is possible to examine a patient carefully, but the doctor cannot see the extent of the microscopic damage within the nervous system. It is also not possible to determine whether the damage to the nerve is due to excess tissue swelling or to scarring. If the damage is due to tissue swelling, as is invariably the case in the first attacks of this disorder, one can confidently expect the condition to recover virtually completely. This is why doctors tend to be somewhat diffident about whether the condition is going to improve rapidly or not. The doctor is unlikely to be dogmatic but will tend to make the patient and relatives accept that over a period of some weeks it will become obvious whether the symptoms are worsening or remaining static.

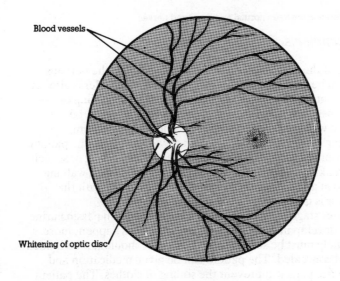

Fig 14 The back of the eye showing the optic disc

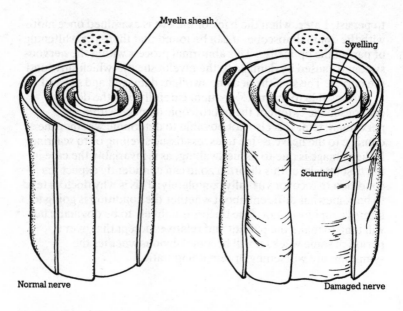

Fig 15 Difference between normal and damaged nerves

Other symptoms

Any part of the nerve-conducting pathways within the nervous system can be affected, and as well as the visual problems already outlined, patients tend to complain of numbness, tingling or altered sensations in hands, arms, legs or feet. This can be associated with weakness and/or clumsiness of movement. Depending on the particular nerve pathways affected, the patient can be troubled with giddiness or difficulty and slurring of speech. As the weakness develops, a patient may have to use a walking stick, and at a late stage walking may become so difficult that a wheelchair is necessary.

At a later stage, the patient may have difficulty in passing urine and may develop incontinence. If the latter does happen, more medical help must be sought, and the matter should not be hidden away and concealed. The patient can be given medication and incontinence pads will prevent the soiling of clothes. The patient and his relatives will also be instructed about the problems of a urinary tract infection and the need to obtain early treatment for this disease.

Informing the patient

This pattern of an initial attack which may well start with blurring of vision or numbness of hands or feet, and progress steadily to a state of considerable restriction of mobility, is a very worrying thing. One of the problems facing the doctor is at what point to discuss the problem in depth with the patient. Most patients feel, I think, they should have been told at an early stage that they were suffering from multiple sclerosis. I would tend to agree with them, but would add that I do not think one should ever tell a patient that he is so affected unless one is certain. It is possible that he can have an attack of painful blurred vision which may last for some weeks, but thereafter experience no further problems. I think in that case it would be quite unnecessary to tell the patient that he is suffering from multiple sclerosis. In the same way, if a patient has an attack of weakness, numbness or giddiness and the condition resolves satisfactorily, he should not be labelled as suffering from this disorder. However, if a patient suffers from multiple attacks of neurological problems, disseminated in time and throughout the nervous system, the diagnosis is really not in doubt.

In this case I think the doctor needs to spend time with his patient, explaining the nature of the disorder in detail and also making very certain that the patient does not feel that his condition will rapidly deteriorate, because this is not so.

Patients tend to think this way because everyone loves the dramatic. It is not of the slightest interest to most people to see somebody fit, happy, healthy and leading an active life and to be told that they suffer from multiple sclerosis. They are unlikely to believe it and it affords them little in the way of dramatic interest. On the other hand, tell them of somebody severely disabled, having to give up their job, and being confined to a wheelchair, and at once most people are interested and will remember it. This means that there are probably quite a few people you know who may well have had attacks of multiple sclerosis in the past, but who lead happy and healthy lives and neither wish nor need to discuss their disease.

Avoiding an attack

The initial and the subsequent attacks may well be precipitated by unusual fatigue, infection, becoming very cold, or as a result of an accident or an allergic reaction. Obviously, there is no way of preventing the first attack, but once the disease has been diagnosed, it is possible to avoid extremes of activity. I am all for people leading as active a life as possible, but at the same time I think it is sensible to follow the sort of ideas that one's mother offered, about wrapping up well and keeping warm in cold weather, not exposing oneself significantly to the chances of a severe cold or sore throat by going into a very crowded smoky atmosphere in the winter or exercising oneself to the point of total exhaustion. On the other hand, I would not suggest that one limits one's activity to any great extent, because there seems little point in going to extremes to prevent a possible attack which may never occur anyway.

Emotional symptoms

As well as the physical symptoms which I have outlined, there are also emotional ones linked with this disorder.

Depression
Inevitably, with such a chronic and relapsing disease the patient is likely to feel significantly depressed on first learning of the problem. He is also likely to wonder whether his feeling of tiredness is due to the disorder or simply to his general feeling of anxiety and depression. This is where a talk with a sympathetic doctor can be of tremendous help. In the main one cannot be exact about this sort of thing, but at least the patient can discuss his feelings.

However, instead of feeling depressed, some patients seem to be happier than one would expect. Whether this is due to the disorder, or to their ability to come to terms with it, is not clear.

Sexual problems
Another significant psychological problem affecting patients is in sexual relationships. As multiple sclerosis is a neurological problem, and the nerves to the bladder and penis can be affected, it is not surprising that men suffer from an increased degree of impotence. Women are also affected because the nerve pathways involved in sexual arousal and orgasm can be damaged.

Patients and doctors are often diffident about discussing these problems, but if a patient is worried about these matters, he should discuss the matter with his doctor. If he would find this too embarrassing, he should write to the Committee of Sexual Problems of the Disabled (SPOD).

The Multiple Sclerosis Society

It is worth joining the Multiple Sclerosis Society. This is dedicated to helping the sufferers from this disorder. There may well be a group of members of the Society in your area who can discuss the problems of the disorder with you in a far more helpful way than if you were to talk them over with your doctor. I hope this is not because we are lacking in sympathy and understanding, but because fellow sufferers have a personal and practical knowledge of the ups and downs of the disorder which we can only perceive from the outside. The need for counselling in such a condition is enormous, and one of the deficiencies of the National Health Service is that such a facility is not available on any large scale.

Coping with multiple sclerosis

However, before becoming too philosophical I will return to the immediate problems of how one deals with the disorder. Unfortunately, there is no specific treatment for this condition. The best advice that a sufferer is likely to get from the doctor during an acute attack is to rest, the degree of which will depend upon the severity of the symptoms. Total bed rest is unlikely to be implemented. What would be suggested instead would be regulated activity to suit the degree of disability. During an acute attack corticotrophin drugs may be injected, to reduce the tissue swelling. They do not have, as far as is known, a direct effect on the actual disease process, but if, for instance, the swelling of the optic nerve is reduced, the visual disturbance can be brought under control at an earlier stage than would have otherwise occurred. The use of these injections over a long period is of no value because the long-term effects of the disease are due to the scarring of the nerve tissue, which cannot be healed. The use of other forms of treatment is regarded by the medical profession as generally worthless. This, of course, poses problems for the patient, and anxious relatives. The patient feels that he should receive some form of treatment. Therefore, he is likely to listen to the odd suggestions that he hears about, reads about or sees in popular magazines. As a result, the patient can be advised to embark on all sorts of special diets, and to take all sorts of strange vitamins and supplements. Unfortunately, such treatments have no scientific validity.

There is a variety of suggestions for the chronic sufferer.

Muscle relaxants

At times, the disorder produces attacks of severe and painful muscle spasm and stiffness, in which case the use of muscle relaxants can be of considerable help.

Physiotherapy

This has a limited part to play, but I do feel that a physiotherapist can often be of great help and comfort when a patient is going through a bad patch, by advising how to make the best use of one's muscle power. However, I do not see any great value in a long attendance at such a clinic.

Walking aids

The patient who is having significant difficulty in walking would be well advised to use a stick. It is not a sign of weakness or defeat to make use of such an aid and it can be a reminder to the patient and his colleagues that he has to limit his activity.

Occupational therapy

If the patient's ability to move is becoming more restricted, the general practitioner, with the help of the hospital clinic, should be able to arrange for occupational therapy to help the patient at home or in hospital. Before embarking on such a course, the doctor would obviously do his very best to ensure that the patient is able to continue at work for as long as possible.

Employment

The doctor should discuss the disability and abilities with the patient and his employers, and suggest that when he is feeling well he can work for all or most of the week, but when he is having difficulty, or as the disease progresses, he should be allowed to work on a part-time basis. Such a person is entitled to register as disabled, and this may be an advantage to the employer. One should also, if necessary, make contact with the Social Services

Department to get assistance with transport and to apply for a mobility allowance. A patient confined to home for any length of time is entitled to the services of a home help and Meals On Wheels service if these are available, and it could well be that the health visitor will become actively involved and visit on a regular basis.

Multiple sclerosis is a very variable disorder. The causes are unknown and at present treatment is not specific. The ultimate outcome for each patient cannot be predicted with success.

Fears And Phobias

All of us, however much we may try to conceal it, are frightened of a few or many objects, people or situations. In fact, we would regard it as significantly abnormal if we met somebody who was not frightened of something.

The variation in our different fears is immense. For instance, I enjoy mountaineering, and to be high up on the edge of a cliff with a significant drop below me does not trouble me as long as I am well and truly attached to the mountain! However, a companion sport of caving or potholing does not really appeal at all. I have been underground and through one or two fairly narrow cave systems, but did not enjoy it and would certainly not be prepared to squeeze myself through a narrow tunnel in the dark, with a feeling that I might not be able to get out at the other side or return the way I came. Many people would feel the same, and I think we would be regarded by the general population as being normal. However, if one's fear of an enclosed space is such that one is frightened to enter a lift, the situation suddenly becomes different. One is then starting to behave very differently from the vast majority of one's contemporaries, and would be regarded with some degree of curiosity by others if they knew of this hidden fear.

In this chapter I shall look at some of the fears that affect us and then move on to several types of *phobia*. This word has an ancient derivation from the Greek and refers to the Greek god Phobos. He was able to instil fear and panic in the enemies of the ancient Greeks, and it is these irrational emotions which are the essential elements of a phobia.

Types of anxiety states

Medical jargon describes a patient as suffering from a *phobic anxiety state*. This is in order to distinguish between the specific irrational fears from which a patient suffers, and the general anxiety which a patient may feel. Thus, there are two big groups of anxiety symptoms, the most common being where the patients are generally anxious. However, in this chapter I shall look at those people who suffer from specific anxieties related to particular objects or situations.

Phobic anxiety

The difference between the two types of anxiety states is the specificity of the patient's phobic anxiety state. When able to lead a life that does not bring him face to face with a specific object or situation, all seems well and an interested onlooker would not know of the deep-seated irrational fear that is produced by, for instance, being confined in an enclosed space, seeing a spider or snake, having to go out of doors, and so on. The list of situations which can cause this condition is endless, because any situation or object can cause the fear in different patients.

The causes of anxiety

I think I should start by saying that all of us have some innate fears. These fears, which are present to a minimal extent within us from birth, can be reinforced or suppressed by our early upbringing. If from an early age one is taught that creepy crawly things are nasty and that snakes are slimy, dangerous and to be feared, it is extremely likely that one will grow up with this fear within one. Maybe over the years one forgets all about it.

Fear of spiders and other insects

However, if a child is unlucky enough to find himself suddenly confronted by an unpleasant-looking insect or spider, he may well panic. If the parents are near at hand they are likely to snatch the child away from this fearsome object, and possibly shout or scream. The seed is then sown. The child's impressionable mind has been conditioned, prior to the incident, to the belief that this particular object is unpleasant. Suddenly the fact has been proved. The child now knows that a spider, for instance, is an object to be feared and will do his best to avoid any future confrontations.

It can well be that the dramatic instance which impresses the fear on the child has nothing to do with his parents. They may be sensible, reasonable people who are quite unworried by, say, spiders or snakes. Instead, he might have schoolfriends who have this sort of fear and who are able to impress it on him because

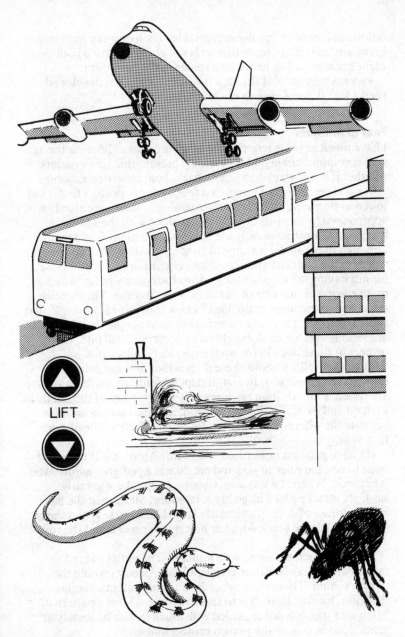

Fig 16 Some of the objects and creatures which create phobias

unfortunately he is equally suggestable. Then one day he comes home and tells his parents that he is not going to have a bath that night because he has just seen a spider in the bathroom.

Parents may scoff at the idea but once a child has developed such a fear it is not easy to eradicate it quickly.

Fear of animals

I have dwelt at some length on spiders and snakes because this is a very common phobia and is so widely present that one wonders whether it is not almost an innate part of our inherited makeup.

What is certainly not innate is a fear of dogs or cats. I find it sad to see some young children run screaming to their parents when approached by our two dogs, walking along with their tails wagging. Almost invariably the parents are equally frightened, although they usually manage to conceal it with a mixture of angry words to the children and sometimes equally angry words to me for not having my dogs under control. I suppose what makes the matter worse is that one of our dogs is an Alsatian. The fact that she is one of the most timid dogs I know convinces few people that she is harmless. There is a basic fear in most people that Alsatians are vicious and, given the slightest opportunity, will bite. Only owners of these dogs know what a complete fallacy that is.

The other fallacy about these dogs is that they are totally devoted to one person. In fact, it depends entirely on the way they are raised. Our Alsatian bitch regards any member of the family as a friend and owner, although undoubtedly she favours my wife because she offered her the most love and affection during her first year.

If I have gone on rather long about this Alsatian it is because I want to compare her to you and me. She is a pedigree animal who is nervous. When she was a very young puppy she was fairly savagely attacked by a large black labrador. Since then she has been terrified of dogs, particularly large black ones. When she is faced with a large black dog, her hair stands on end and she runs away very fast.

It is very much the same with humans. The initial triggering factor, which may be rational or irrational, persists within the person's mind. Thereafter, when he finds himself in a similar situation, his first instinct is to run away fast. This is a pattern of behaviour which is not regarded with much favour by society in general, so how does the person protect himself?

Coping with specific fears

The most sensible course is to avoid the situation or object. Therefore, if you are frightened of enclosed spaces you do not get into a lift; if you are frightened of being up a mountain, or looking over the edge of a building, you do not expose yourself to this fear. In these sorts of situations it is usually quite easy to prevent the fear building up by avoiding it. However, there are some patients who find that the specific fear or object so intrudes into their daily life that they are unable to lead the life that they or their family would wish. In this case they obviously need help and treatment. This is in direct contrast to the previous cases, where the person does not feel that he is ill, and therefore has no wish to avail himself of any help.

Before moving on further I should perhaps say that the psychoanalytical view of phobias is rather more complex than the simple scheme I have outlined. The classic case which was described by Freud many years ago was of a boy called Little Hans, who had a fear of being bitten by a horse. When Freud investigated the matter in considerable detail by analysing the boy's behaviour, he came to the conclusion that the boy had displaced an underlying anxiety for his father onto a horse. In simple terms he saw them both as big, strong and menacing. I find this sort of approach fascinating, though not always convincing.

More complex phobias

In the original definition of a phobia I stated that it was a specific anxiety linked either to an object or a situation. The objects I have mentioned are insects, reptiles and the like, but it can equally be any other form of object. Sometimes the nature of the object can easily be linked with the phobia. For instance, a patient can be afraid to be near a knife because he fears that if he handles it he will be impelled to injure himself with it. This is a complex psychological situation in which a patient is going to need expert help to settle the emotional problem that almost certainly has been troubling him for a long time.

Common phobias
The phobias which tend to cause the most trouble are fear of

enclosed spaces (claustrophobia), heights, darkness, loneliness, crowds and fear of open spaces (agoraphobia). In fact, if one is a Greek scholar, one can produce a whole series of impressive-sounding Greek names for virtually any phobia one would like to mention. However, there are some phobias which are very common.

Agoraphobia

Firstly there is the problem of the housebound housewife. Usually the story is that of a youngish mother with a baby or toddler, probably living in a newish housing estate and feeling rather lonely and depressed following the birth of the child. She has recovered her strength and energy but may well be somewhat tired, anxious and suffering from sleepless nights. She finds the effort of leading an ordinary life troublesome and the difficulties of going out to do her shopping and talking to friends even more so. After a while, the effort and strain of going out and having to make decisions in the local shops becomes too much for her.

In each case, something has happened to cause the condition. Problems at home, problems with the in-laws, problems with her husband, worries and fears about her child, difficulties with finance, fears of her husband being made redundant, or a combination of all these, add to her own basically somewhat anxious personality so that eventually she is unable to leave the house. The thought of going out on her own into a social gathering is so bad that she becomes housebound. Left at home she is well able to manage, but force her to go outside and she will go hot and cold, feel her pulse and heart race, feel weak and trembly and think that her legs will collapse. It is a hardhearted strong-minded person who can force such a woman out of the house. Almost invariably she will stay inside. Usually with coaxing she is able to go outside and do her shopping when she is accompanied by a child or adult.

This causes a lot of disruption in the household. The child has to stay away from school in order to allow his mother to go shopping, or the husband has to leave work early, or take time off from work, in order to allow her to lead a reasonably normal life. I think this is intolerable for a family unit, and they should seek advice and help.

School phobia

Another common anxiety is one which usually affects early

teenage children. This is known as school phobia. The usual story is that a pleasant, somewhat shy, reasonably intelligent child has just left primary school and is worried and anxious. It may be that the child's friends are not going to the same new school, or that this school is already known to the child or the parents as being in a rough, tough area. It could be that the journey is longer than the child has had to experience before and that the bus route is not known to him. Perhaps the mother has recently recovered from a serious illness, or is basically an anxious worrying person who shows her fear of the child going to a new school. As a result, the child may attend the new school for a week or so and then suffer a series of minor illnesses. These keep the child away from school for longer than one would expect and then finally he stops going to school altogether. The child, when questioned, will explain that he is terrified of going to school. However, when asked to give specific reasons about the problems at the school, he is almost always unable to produce any actual information. Nearly always in these situations it is not the fear of going to school that is the problem, but the fear of leaving home.

In other words, the agoraphobia and the school phobia are very similar. In both cases somebody is bound to the house. In the first example, it is the house as a structure and entity which gives security to the young mother, and in the second it is the mother's presence in the house and the fear of leaving her which prevents the child from going out to school.

One could endlessly describe other phobic anxiety states but I hope the descriptions I have given of the fears of insects and animals, and fears of leaving the home, are a sufficiently reasonable representation of the very varied pattern of this problem. In all these cases one can see a mixture of reasonable and irrational fears, a pattern of striving to overcome the fear, or a complete inability to deal with it at all. There is an obsessional pattern about some of these fears which is very evident in some patients' personalities, but this is certainly not the case in all people suffering from this sort of disorder.

Treatment

How then can such people be helped? Firstly I think one should say that if the specific fear is not sufficiently disabling and

73

troublesome to the patient and to those around him, to make him feel he needs help, then no help need be offered. It would seem unrealistic to me to suggest to someone living in a flat part of the country, and unlikely in his general life ever to have to go up a high mountain, that his fear of heights should be cured.

Treatment or help needs to be offered when there is a disruption to the person's life, or there is significant disruption to those living near the patient. Often family or friends can offer comfort and support, but at the same time they can make the situation worse by accepting it and not making the patient face his phobia. Alternatively, they can make the situation worse by ridicule.

Seeing the general practitioner

I feel that anybody who has a specific fear should see his general practitioner early. I would hope that once he realised that this was not just a simple problem but a significantly disabling condition, he would set time aside for a full investigation. He would need to know something about his patient's childhood and upbringing, and have some idea of the family history and occupational history. He would have to convince the patient that his is a relatively common problem, that he is not going mad and that there would be no question of his being admitted to a mental hospital.

The immediate treatment a general practitioner is likely to offer is comfort and reassurance, possibly together with mild anxiety-relieving drugs. He might prescribe others to specifically stop the heart racing when the patient is faced with a situation of acute anxiety.

At the same time, I think the doctor has to adopt the role of the firm friendly challenger. It is no good for the patient, or the family, to allow the child to stay away from school, or the mother to remain in the house. Therefore, I feel that at an early stage the expert help of a psychiatric team is needed in order to try to overcome the difficulties.

Psychiatric help

A psychiatrist or psychiatric team would approach the problem in the same way as a sympathetic general practitioner. However, because the psychiatrist has more time and better facilities, the patient is able to describe his symptoms in greater detail, paying particular attention to his previous life and upbringing, family history, occupational history, and a whole range of other facts which may have caused the problem.

Depending on the type of clinic, it is possible that a psycho-analytical approach may be offered. I think, and there will be psychiatric colleagues who will disagree with me, that this is time-consuming, lengthy and to my mind usually not appropriate to this problem.

I believe that the best way to deal with a phobic anxiety state is through a team approach. I would include in the team, as well as the psychiatrist and his psychologically trained colleagues, the general practitioner, the family, and school or employer, as appropriate.

Of course it is sensible to try to find out why a patient is frightened of a specific object or situation. At times this is easy and at times very difficult. However, even when one does know why, it often does not improve the situation at all when it is explained to the patient, who agrees with the logical reasoning, but is still unable to face the object or situation. Then it is appropriate to use the dual technique of initiating relaxation on the one hand and a *deconditioning programme* on the other.

Deconditioning programme

I will explain in some detail this form of medical jargon describing a form of behaviour therapy. To take a simple example, the patient has a fear of insects and, in particular, spiders. A clinical psychologist will find out from the patient what type of spider in what sort of situation produces the greatest fear. For instance, the patient may say the thought of a large black furry spider in a small room with him would be absolutely intolerable. On the other hand, the thought of a small spider in an open space would not cause him any worry at all.

The clinical psychologist and the patient then construct what is known as a hierarchy of situations. The hierarchy starts with a simple non-threatening situation, such as talking about spiders. The next situation might be looking at a picture of a spider, which produces mild anxiety. Gradually one builds up the series until the patient accepts that the final stage would be to confront a spider or to actually tolerate a spider in his hand.

A list of situations has now been drawn up, which the patient and psychologist agree they are going to work through. The situations may number 10 or 12.

Relaxation

At the same time, the patient will be taught methods of relaxation which will be performed each time the patient attends the clinic. The object of the treatment then is to make the patient visit the clinic to practice the relaxation exercises. Once he is fully relaxed and can maintain the relaxation, he will be confronted with the first situation. Gradually the patient progresses, being able to tolerate more situations, and relying on the help, reassurance and support of the clinical psychologist, until finally the patient can cope with the final stage. It is at this moment, if he can maintain it, that he is cured.

This sounds easy, but as you can imagine, it is neither simple nor straightforward and there are many stumbling starts and stops, retreats and advances before the patient discovers that all his fears and worries were groundless and it is possible to lead a normal life which includes the feared object or situation.

Implosion therapy

The use of a deconditioning and relaxation technique is obviously time-consuming and at times one offers virtually the opposite form of therapy. This is known as *implosion* or *swamping therapy*. This means that instead of carefully working through a hierarchy, one discusses the whole situation in detail with the patient and his relatives. I think this is by far the best way to tackle a school phobic problem, if one sees the child at an early stage. To my mind this is one of the few childhood psychiatric emergencies. I am always pleased to see a child who is refusing to go to school in the early stages of the anxiety, when I aim to get the child back to school at once, before the pattern of non-attendance becomes imprinted on the child's mind.

In a psychiatric clinic one has to mobilise all one's forces to overcome the fear. The key members of the child's school, such as the headmaster and schoolteacher, together with the school Welfare Officer and the School Attendance Officer, should discuss the matter with both parents and the general practitioner. Once one has got all their support, one explains to the child that although all of us would be happy not to go to school, we all have to do it, even though she might think it a fearful business. It might also be explained that we have to go in order to acquire a suitable level of knowledge to cope with the civilised society in which we live. The child is spoken to in a firm, friendly, sympathetic manner and it is made very clear that one means what one says. Having then mobilised all the forces, the child goes to school the following day. Once at the school, it is vital that the headmaster and the teachers are prepared to accept the initial tremendous fear and anxiety which the child will manifest. However, very often once the child is away from home and back in school all the fears evaporate, and he suddenly finds that the school is not the dreaded place that he believed it to be.

It is because these fears build up so quickly that it is so necessary to act swiftly in these cases. I feel very strongly about this because I find, as a practising child psychiatrist myself, that it is dreadful to see a child who has been off school for perhaps three or six months, and is now so convinced that he cannot return there that in fact *it is* virtually impossible to get such a child back. The only way to deal with such a situation then is for the child to leave home and enter a residential clinic with an attached school. This seems to me to be a very unfortunate way of dealing with a phobic situation which, if tackled in the early days, could have been resolved very successfully.

Other forms of treatment

Another way of dealing with the problems of a phobic anxiety state is through hypnosis, although I have had little experience of patients treated in this way. Alternatively, a very strict specific drug regime can be prescribed. In the past, the ultimate form of treatment for somebody who was totally disabled by the condition would have been an operation to the front of the brain. This operation, known as a *pre frontal leucotomy*, used to be very much in vogue for the treatment of severe obsessional and depressive states, but has now fallen into disuse and it is extremely unlikely that it would be performed on a patient now.

Of more value to a patient suffering from a phobic state is the modern hospital approach which I have already outlined. In addition to this, many psychiatric hospitals have a day hospital unit. Here, patients suffering from a variety of phobias can be taught various skills and techniques to overcome their disabilities. They are also retrained in social skills, such as how to use a bank, so that they can take a much more active part in the society in which they live.

Finally, I should repeat that all of us normally suffer from fears. Some people have specific phobias which do not cause trouble, but for those who do, such treatment as that outlined above is now available throughout the country and is effective if followed. The general practitioner and the psychiatrist are there to help, but it is only possible for them to provide such help if the patient is prepared to accept the initial difficulties of combating the fear. Once started on the treatment pattern the patient will usually improve so significantly that he will wonder why he did not come earlier.

Parkinson's Disease

In medicine there is a variety of diseases which are named after the man who originally described them. This is usually because his description was so clinically clear and precise that thereafter his name was always linked with the disease. Such is the case with the disease discussed in this chapter.

Dr James Parkinson was a general practitioner in London, who described this condition in 1870. It is a disorder which usually affects people over the age of 60. About 80,000 people suffer from it in this country. Its onset is slow and insidious and unfortunately there is no specific cure, although the condition can be relieved considerably.

Symptoms

Tremor

The disorder begins with a tremor which typically occurs in one hand at first. This tremor is often referred to as pill rolling, because the movements of the fingers and thumb suggest that the person is rolling material between them. The tremor is usually regular, at a rate of between four and eight movements per second. Initially, the patient is able to control the tremor by conscious effort but can only do so manually. For instance, if he has a tremor of his left hand and the right hand is not affected, he can grasp the left hand with the right and hide the movement, but unfortunately he is unable to obliterate it fully. The tremor is worse when the patient is at rest, but often it is reduced when he is moving the affected limb, and disappears completely when the patient is asleep.

Muscular rigidity

At a later stage the other main symptoms develop. The first is when the patient develops muscular rigidity, and if this affects the leg muscles, as it is likely to do, there is a problem in walking. The rigidity of the muscles can be demonstrated by a clinical sign known as *cog wheel rigidity*. If the patient who has a tremor in his left hand also feels some rigidity, he will find that when he bends his wrist, he will do so in a jerky manner reminiscent of a cog wheel.

If the muscles of the legs are similarly affected, the patient will have difficulty in walking. The easy fluid confident motion of the legs goes. Most of us take walking for granted, and forget what a complex balancing act it is. Put this book down for a few moments and walk round the room and then sit down again. You will notice that you stood up with ease, were able to walk round the furniture without any difficulty, could turn without a struggle and then swing back into your chair.

However, this ease of movement tends to go as the patient with Parkinson's disease steadily deteriorates over the years. He can no longer stand up quickly, and when he walks his legs tend to jerk forward because of the cog wheel effect. Without even thinking, when walking we fling our arms forward and backwards to counterbalance our legs. If we have difficulties with our legs we move our arms more. However, a patient suffering from Parkinson's disease will have difficulty in moving his arms as well as his legs. The outcome of this is that he will walk slowly and at times will tend to shuffle along because of the problems with movement, rigidity and balance.

Facial rigidity

Because the rigidity and tremor can attack other muscle groups, the muscles of the face are also affected in some patients. This causes them to have a mask-like look. This is the other major symptom.

When a person talks he constantly moves his eyebrows, forehead, nose and cheek muscles to convey moods, feelings and expressions. He is able to register emotions on his face too, such as affection, pleasure or anger. The patient with Parkinson's disease, however, is unable to convey this variety of expression and instead wears a stony look. This is most unfortunate because it needs to be emphasised now, that the patient is mentally and emotionally absolutely normal. He can hear, think, feel, reason and express himself with no difficulty whatsoever. However, his face is unable to convey his moods and feelings as quickly as it might and because the muscles affecting his voice can also be disordered, his speech can be slurred and blurred.

Being unable to convey his emotions can be very frustrating to a patient, and he can become irritable and depressed. He needs considerable help in order to come to terms with this situation.

Dribbling

As a result of these muscular problems, a patient may dribble from his mouth because he is unable to swallow with ease the saliva he produces. He is as embarrassed and annoyed about this as his friends may be, but he has to live with it all the time, whereas they only have to accept it for part of the time. It is very infuriating to be unable to cope with this problem because one cannot move one's arms quickly to remove the excess saliva with a handkerchief.

Manipulative movements

The rigidity and the slowness of movement which affects speech, facial expression and walking is also troublesome in other ways. The patient who has difficulty with fine manipulative movements, will have problems with such activities as writing or dressing.

One of the problems with this condition is that the symptoms vary in severity, therefore leading relatives and friends to believe that the patient is at times pretending. This is not true. There is no doubt that the stress of meeting strangers, or any anxiety, generalized or specific, makes the tremor and rigidity worse. This must be accepted by those who are interested in helping and caring for such a person.

Constipation

Another symptom which can cause trouble is that of constipation. This is not surprising when one considers that it takes a regular, forceful action to empty the bowels. It is therefore important that a patient suffering from this disorder ensures that his bowels do open regularly. However, he must avoid the over-use of laxatives. He should read the chapter on constipation once more and consult his doctor if it is a significant problem. The bladder is not usually affected but occasionally may be, in which case he should seek medical advice as to how best this problem can be resolved.

I have painted the picture at its worst, but do remember that not all patients suffer in such a way and that if the condition is noticed at an early stage, when there is just a tremor in one hand, it can be stabilised with modern drugs, and life made more comfortable than it might otherwise have been.

What causes Parkinson's disease?

Unfortunately, the cause of this disease is not known. Several years ago, some cases were related to a vast epidemic of a brain infection known as *encephalitis lethargica*. This particular infection swept the world in about 1920, and some of the victims of this disorder developed Parkinson-like symptoms some months or years later. The majority of these patients are, of course, no longer alive.

Some Parkinson-like symptoms can be produced by a high dosage of drugs given for some mental disorders. However, this is usually immediately apparent to the doctors dealing with such cases, and the dosage of the drugs reduced, thereby eliminating the troublesome symptoms.

Although the specific cause is unknown, it is known which area and mechanisms of the brain are affected. The disorder is due to a slowly progressive deterioration of certain specific nerve cells situated at the base of the brain. They are present in a portion of the brain known as the *substantia nigra*, so-called because of its dark colour when looked at under a microscope.

This portion of the brain is responsible for controlling muscle action. The exact way in which the system works is not known but if you can imagine the brain as a vast computer, with the nerve cells stimulating or depressing muscle activity, one can understand that there must be some outside control to stop muscles from being overstimulated and contracting, or becoming too relaxed and not moving at all. There is a very delicate balance which keeps the muscles at the right tension. If this balance is upset, as this disorder shows, a pattern of rigidity and tremor develops.

The specific reason for this was discovered in the 1960s, and it is due to the lack in the brain of a chemical substance known as *dopamine*. For reasons not known, the substantia nigra in this condition fails to produce an adequate quantity of dopamine, resulting in the symptoms. Because the nerve cells are damaged, it is not possible to cure the condition. At present, damaged nerve cells cannot be repaired, and the body has no mechanism for dealing with this situation either. If one cuts a nerve in, for instance, an arm or foot, the cells in the spinal cord, together with all the other cells responsible for the formation of a nerve, are able to very slowly regrow. If, however, the actual nerve cell itself is damaged, the body is unable to repair it. Unfortunately, modern medicine is unable to help.

There is no specific hereditary factor in Parkinson's disease, but it is possible that there is some small famial disposition so that it is slightly more common in families where there already is a case present.

Treatment

Anticholinergic drugs

When I qualified as a medical student, about 25 years ago, Parkinson's disease was helped to some extent by a variety of drugs known as *anticholinergics*. Some patients found these very helpful but unfortunately they did not help everyone. The dosage had to be adjusted for each patient in order to obtain the maximum duration of effect. It usually meant taking them three or four times a day, and one had to accept the side effects of dryness of the mouth, blurring of vision and possible constipation or difficulty in passing urine. Some people overreact to medication and this is particularly so as one becomes older. As a result, some elderly patients would become somewhat confused or dizzy when taking large doses. However, these drugs were very helpful and still continue to be used.

Surgery

In the 1960s, specific surgery to the brain was undertaken and this was a great advance. Because in this condition the brain damages a part of itself, the neurosurgeons damaged a further portion of the brain nearby, using special probes. This meant the inbalance of muscle action was to a large extent overcome, and patients obtained significant relief. However, the surgery was complex and though helpful, was not without its problems.

Today, surgical treatment is usually reserved for the younger patient in good health, whose disability only affects one side of his body and who does not have difficulty with speech or walking. It is the most effective method of relieving tremor, but unfortunately its effect on muscular rigidity is not as great.

83

Dopaminergic drugs

The basic deficit in this condition is the lack of the chemical dopamine, but during the last 10 years or so it has been possible to produce a drug known as *levodopa,* which replaces the dopamine not present in the brain of these patients. It is taken by mouth in the form of dopaminergic tablets, which give almost complete relief of symptoms in about 20% of patients. In fact, most people taking them show some improvement, although it may well take a considerable time for the maximum benefit to be noticed. If you or a friend or relative is prescribed one of these drugs, you must be prepared to persevere for at least six months before you gain the maximum benefit. The difficulty and slowness of movements are the symptoms which respond best. This is good because it is these symptoms which are often the most distressing. Therefore, the rigidity, which is the cause of the problem, can be relieved significantly. The tremor, however, is usually the last symptom to improve and may not improve at all.

Dosage

The dosage of the tablets containing the levodopa depends upon the particular patient's response. There is tremendous variation in the number of tablets a patient needs and the number he can accept without significant side effects. Some patients may take 10 to 15 tablets a day, whereas others may only need two or four. The doctor and the patient should work out a scheme whereby the tablets are steadily increased over a period of two to three weeks until a reasonable dosage is obtained, which is not causing significant distress to the patient.

Side effects

The side effects of levodopa are nausea and vomiting if taken on an empty stomach, and the patient may also feel dizzy or faint. These side effects are reduced if the levodopa is combined with a substance known as decarboxylase inhibitor. These combined tablets are more commonly used nowadays because the additive helps to increase the effect of the levodopa as well as to reduce the side effects.

Unfortunately, another side effect of the simple or combined drug is the involuntary movement of the face or limbs. Obviously, this is the last thing one wants to produce in a patient who is already having muscular problems. Although these side effects may develop quite early, they can also appear at a later stage. At either time, the dosage will have to be reduced.

However, when taking these drugs, it is quite normal for the urine to become dark and discoloured. This is caused by the levodopa being excreted from the body.

Other helpful drugs

As well as the anticholinergic and the dopamine replacement drugs, some other drugs are used which have a similar action to dopamine. I will not go into detail about them here but a specialist clinic may use them if they find them to be more effective than dopamine replacement therapy.

The basic rule with the treatment of Parkinson's disease is that one should use the drugs in a careful manner, and be prepared to persevere with them for a considerable time in order to see that the maximum effect is being derived. If side effects occur, the dosage should be reduced at once to a level which does not produce those side effects. Obviously, in order to balance the medical treatment effectively the patient, doctor and relatives should establish a good liason so that they can discuss what is happening and between them monitor the condition properly.

Coping with Parkinson's disease

I have now looked at the treatment that is available for this condition, and suggested a variety of drugs which can be helpful. However, the drugs are unlikely to completely relieve all the symptoms, and will probably leave a patient with some degree of disability, be it tremor, rigidity or difficulty in movement. He has to live with the problem and with himself, and therefore it is important that he is prepared to help himself as best he can. Certain simple measures can well make a considerable improvement in his way of life.

Finding fellow sufferers

First I would suggest that any patient suffering from this disorder should join the Parkinson's Disease Society. This has been in operation now for over 10 years and produces a series of most helpful booklets on the condition. There are local groups scattered throughout the country and if there is not one in your area, it could well be that having joined the nearest one, and read the literature, you or your family could be interested in trying to start such a group yourselves. I would suggest that you join the Society as soon as possible and purchase the various booklets which are produced. You will find that they cover much the same ground that I have tried to do in this chapter, but they are written by experts with more knowledge and experience than I have.

Exercise

I think it is important that you try to keep as active, and lead as interesting a life, as possible. As I mentioned at the beginning of this chapter, a patient suffering from this condition may well be over the age of 60 and retired. Because of the difficulty with movement it could be tempting to sit back and do nothing. This is wrong. It is far better to try to exercise as much as one reasonably can. A walk taken each day in the patient's area will be of benefit to him physically and emotionally. However, he should always walk in sensible well-fitting shoes because, as has been mentioned earlier, walking and balancing can be a problem and it would be foolish for him to fall over because his shoes did not fit. Anyone worried about walking should carefully plan a route first. This may be necessary until the patient has confidence. Later, if the patient has difficulty, someone should accompany him. He should do his best to walk on his own but if he needs a friendly hand under his arm, he should be certain that his walking colleague understands his difficulties, and does not try to pull or drag him along.

As well as the social and emotional benefits that walking gives, it obviously helps the muscles in the legs. Other troublesome rigid muscles should also be exercised, wherever they are. For example, the fingers and wrists, elbows or shoulders should be bent and flexed for five or ten minutes once or twice a day. However, the patient should not be too obsessional about this, and should not overtire himself. Instead, he should remember that he is doing this for his own benefit and so should find his own limit.

Coping with dribbling

Earlier on I mentioned the problem of dribbling saliva, which is really infuriating. It is possible to prescribe tablets which dry up the mouth, but most patients find that this produces even more discomfort. If a patient can practice swallowing, he might be able to help himself control the problem of excess salivation by learning to consciously swallow at reasonably frequent intervals.

Manoeuvrability in the home

Furniture

It is important that beds and chairs are at the right height for a patient. He should experiment with both until he finds a chair which is right for him. If his bed is difficult to get in and out of, then he should consider carefully whether he can afford to buy a new one, or whether he knows anyone who can raise or lower it to an appropriate level. Of course, a simple method would be to put blocks under the bed.

I dislike nylon sheets because I slip around on them, but a patient suffering from this disorder who has difficulty turning might find them ideal, and this is a possible answer to the problem of moving around in bed. The use of a handrail alongside, or an overhead rail, may also help a patient to get in or out of bed or change position while in bed. It will improve the morale and self-respect of the patient if he is able to do these things for himself.

Adapting rooms

The problems of moving and manipulating items around the house should be looked at in relation to adapting the bathroom, the toilet, the stairs and the kitchen. This is an area which has improved considerably over the past few years. The local Social Services Department should be able to help, but more specialised help can be obtained from the Disabled Living Foundation, which produces pamphlets and literature and can offer advice on the problems of living with a disability at home or outside. For instance, a patient can be helped significantly with gardening, if that is his hobby, by learning to use the range of modern gardening instruments designed specially for the disabled.

Driving

Finally, I should mention that if the disability is of any significance, and the patient drives a car, he must inform the authorities of his problem. This may mean that he needs his doctor's authority before he is eligible for a driving licence. Obviously, he should stop driving altogether if he finds it impossible, because he is then a risk on the road, not only to himself, but to others, and he would not be covered by his insurance policy.

If this chapter has seemed somewhat depressing, I am sorry. I have been dealing with a disease, the cause of which is not known, and the treatment of which, though it has improved dramatically over the last few years, is still not fully effective.

I do think, however, that there is significant hope for the future. Research continues apace and I would imagine that over the next 10 years the pattern of treatment will improve steadily, as it has done during the past decade. Therefore, remember if this condition affects you, to remain as active as you reasonably can but avoid becoming too fatigued. Accept that you will have your good and bad phases and that if you are affected by some other illness or infection, the condition is almost certainly going to become worse. Do avoid becoming constipated and also do your best not to become overweight. If you are having difficulty with your muscles the best way to help them is to make certain that they do not have to move more weight around than is necessary.

Patients' Rights

Under The National Health Service

The National Health Service (NHS) has been the main supplier of medical services in this country since 1948. Of course, anyone living in this country can seek private medical treatment if he wishes to do so, in which case he has a responsibility to work with his private doctor in exactly the same way as he would work with his solicitor or architect. I do not intend to go into the problems, benefits or difficulties of private practice in any detail in this chapter, because the vast majority of people obtain their medical treatment under the National Health Service. Under the NHS Act, every person living in this country is entitled to medical treatment. As soon as one has made this statement, of course, one is then forced to qualify it. The treatment is not free, in that one has to pay for it out of one's taxes, and there are various charges for the different items that one obtains when one is unwell, such as the prescription charge. One also has to pay for various appliances, spectacles and dentures. However, undoubtedly the actual act of seeing a doctor, being examined, being investigated, having a diagnosis made and the subsequent treatment at home or in hospital, is free. One has only to go abroad and be faced with the very high charges for a consultation to realise what a tremendous system we have.

There is, however, no statement in the NHS Act that the treatment will be provided instantaneously, will be always perfect and will provide a total cure. One of the constant conflicts which faces doctors is that we live in an age of unreal expectations. This is a plastic age in which people expect instant packaged service and yet at the same time hope that the article will have the quality and beauty of one which is handmade by a craftsman. If one is looking for instant magic one cannot expect long-standing and long-lasting quality.

It has become also increasingly fashionable these days to attack the medical profession. We are regarded as overbearing, autocratic, unprepared to communicate, uninterested in our patients, only looking for money, doing our best to keep people out of the profession and often not even interested in offering the best form of treatment. I find these sorts of attacks sad and usually do not bother to take issue with them because I generally feel that the people launching the attack have got some personal, though perhaps hidden, problem which they have had difficulty with over the years. On the other hand, I know that there are members of my own profession, as there are in all professions and trades, who do function badly and to whom all the attacks that I have just mentioned apply. Equally, I would accept that there are times when I do not offer anything like as good a service as I should because I am functioning inefficiently on that particular day. I hope that most of the time I offer an efficient and sympathetic service, and I am sure that this applies to the vast majority of my colleagues.

In fact, we all enjoy attacking the services that are offered to us. I could just as easily complain at the way the garage services my car, or the way the television rental service deals with my television set, but I won't do so because in the main I believe that most people tend to do their best. At the same time, I can tell graphic and sometimes amusing stories of the ways in which I have been misled, taken for a ride and generally done down over the years.

I hope I have now offered some sort of defence for my colleagues, who I feel are generally conscientious, hard-working and devoted.

Registering with a general practitioner

In order to obtain treatment from a NHS general practitioner it is necessary to register with him by filling in a form. If one was born in this country, a small form would have been produced at the registration of one's birth. Normally, one's parents would take this to their own doctor, who would complete it, and from that moment one would be registered with a general practitioner.

If one has been out of the country for some while, or has been in the Armed Forces, or for one reason or another does not have a general practitioner, one can go to the doctor of one's choice and ask to register. The general practitioner has the right to accept or refuse.

Most doctors organise their practice lists in a geographical manner. In a large crowded city one will find that most general practitioners set a practice boundary of about 2 miles (3km) or so around their surgery. In the country, the area an individual practice covers will be considerably larger, with doctors in some of the more remote rural areas prepared to travel 15 miles (24km) or more from their village surgeries.

Doctors usually like to register a whole family on their list. They find it is not a good idea to have the husband on one list, and the mother and children on another. Of course, this can lead to difficulties if a patient feels strongly that he does not want to change doctors on marriage, and in most practices a flexible attitude is adopted. However, from the doctor's point of view, it is obviously better to offer a service to a whole family, when one can get to know them over the years, and develop an understanding of their problems.

Choosing a doctor

How should a patient choose a doctor if, for instance, he has moved into a new area? I would suggest that he asks his near neighbours which doctors there are in the town, and what sort of services they operate. Nowadays, most doctors work in group practices. In the group each doctor may look after his own list of patients or the group may share the patients, so that although the patient may register with one doctor, he can be seen by any of them. There is also an increasing number of women doctors in practice today.

Surgery times
The prospective patient should find out the times of the surgeries in order to ensure that he is able to attend them without too much disruption. Doctors are increasingly tending to do afternoon and early evening sessions, rather than the old pattern of having no clinic session in the afternoon and doing a long evening session instead.

Appointment systems
Some doctors have a practice with no appointments, but most doctors do now run an appointment system. If a patient has strong ideas about one or other of these methods, he should see if there is a practice in his area which operates the sort of system which appeals to him.

I have been involved in practices running appointment systems for some years now, and have found that as long as it operates in a flexible manner the system helps both doctor and patient. In the practice in which I work, there are five doctors. Each morning one doctor does not have any appointments, and therefore is able to see any patient who needs to be seen urgently but has not made an appointment.

Other practices arrange gaps throughout the morning and afternoon sessions, so that the patients who arrive without an appointment and feel they need to be seen can be slotted in. Certainly I think that any patient who feels he must be seen that day should be seen. If, however, the problem is not particularly urgent or serious, I think it only fair that the doctor, having dealt with the immediate symptoms, should suggest to the patient that he makes a further appointment, at which the matter can be dealt with in a more efficient manner.

Every practice has a little clutch of patients who will always function in their own way, whatever the system. It seems to me that it is a part of human behaviour which has to be accepted and we well know that no matter how we organise systems, some patients, however intelligent and competent in other ways, will never be prepared to conform to them. With some we just turn a blind eye and let them run the system to suit their own needs, but others who are obviously manipulating us, sometimes in an unpleasant manner, are confronted with their behaviour and told that if they want to remain as patients in the practice it would be better if they accepted the various simple rules laid down by that practice.

The doctor/patient relationship

At times, however, doctors and patients argue. It is usually a personality conflict, though at times the patient may well feel aggrieved because he thinks that the doctor has failed to make the right diagnosis and treat him efficiently. What can the doctor or patient do in these circumstances?

Having signed the initial registration form, both sides have a legal obligation to each other. The doctor undertakes to provide a 24-hour service to the patient, and this includes visiting at home if he feels it is necessary. The patient has a legal obligation not to consult other National Health doctors in the neighbourhood but to remain the patient of one doctor until such time as he feels he wants to officially change.

The patient changing his doctor

If a patient feels that he has not received adequate treatment from his doctor, the simplest way of dealing with the matter is to make an appointment with the doctor concerned, and discuss it with him in detail. If the patient feels that he cannot do this, he should discuss the problem with one of the partners in the practice. If the matter is dealt with at this level, I think that most problems can be solved fairly simply, and both sides are able to learn from the mistakes which have occured. However, the patient may go to any other doctor in the area and ask if he can be accepted as a patient, but not unnaturally, the neighbouring general practitioners tend to be slightly wary about accepting such patients, particularly if the doctor from whom the patient is trying to change is known to be a good, kind and efficient person. However, if he is not so highly regarded then it may be quite easy to change doctors, particularly if it is in an area with a lot of doctors.

The National Health card has to be signed by the new doctor, and if the change is to take place at once, by the preceding doctor as well. If the patient does not have the courage to go into the original doctor and ask him to sign the form of consent to change, he does not have to do so. The patient posts the card to the local office of the Family Practitioner Committee (or its equivalent in Scotland and Northern Ireland) with a note saying that he wishes to change doctors. The card will be returned with a special label inside entitling the patient to change doctors over the next month. If a patient does not do so within this time, this request becomes null and void.

The doctor changing his patient

The process of changing doctors is therefore basically simple, but can cause significant difficulties to both sides. On the doctor's side, if he finds that he can no longer offer the sort of medical treatment he wishes to a patient or family he can write to the Family Practitioner Committee requesting them to remove this patient or family from his list. A letter is then sent to the patient or family, explaining the situation. It is then up to the patients concerned to find another doctor.

In the meantime, until this is effected, the original doctor is under an obligation to treat his patients, and not unnaturally this will cause some embarrassment on both sides.

If the patient is unable to find a new doctor because the local practices will not accept him, there is a legal way of obtaining another doctor. The patient writes to the Family Practitioner Committee and places the problem before them. It is then the duty of the Committee to find a doctor for the patient. If necessary a patient is allocated to a general practitioner who is legally obliged to accept. However, this obligation is not permanent, and if after some months the doctor and patient do not get on, the new doctor is entitled to remove the patient and the family from his list.

Lodging a formal complaint

Every patient has the right, under the 1948 Act, to lodge a formal complaint with the Administrator of the Family Practitioner Committee. He will accept your complaint if he receives it within a reasonable time of the problem arising. If he thought the problem was not too serious, he might try to deal with it in an informal manner, but if he felt that the terms of service as laid down under the Act had been breached, he would arrange a formal hearing.

Both the doctor and the patient present their versions of the situation at the hearing. They are both allowed to be assisted by a friend, who must be neither a paid council nor a solicitor. In the event of the doctor being found in breach of service, the Family Practitioner Committee may fine or admonish him. If the case is regarded as very serious, he may not be allowed to remain in practice as a National Health Service doctor. On the other hand, if the case is not accepted, the doctor has no redress against the patient, although the patient may of course appeal to the Department of Health and Social Security if he feels that he is still in the right.

Treatment of non-British subjects

If one is not normally resident in this country but has come here from overseas, on a visit, or to work, then one is entitled to the benefits of the National Health Service for treatment of illnesses which develop in this country. At the time of going to press, it is likely that regulations will soon be laid before Parliament, which will make any form of medical treatment chargeable. However, illnesses which were present before one arrived in this country are not the responsibility of the National Health Service and treatment for these is provided, if the patient so wishes, privately. The old stories of people flying in from America in order to obtain treatment on the National Health Service are no longer applicable.

Home visits

One of the problems which beset general practice in its early years, after it was instituted in 1948, was the right of the patient to demand that the doctor visited. Quite rightly, many general practitioners felt this was very irksome. Some patients were very demanding, feeling that because they had the right to request a visit, they could do so even for minor problems. In 1966 the Act was altered, so that although the patient, or his relatives or friends on his behalf, are fully entitled to ask the doctor to visit, it is the doctor's responsibility to determine whether it is necessary or not. The onus now is very firmly placed on the doctor, but of course he bears the responsibility if he fails to visit when necessary.

Speaking on the telephone

Very often conflicts arise because of the way messages are transmitted. The telephone is not an easy instrument to handle, lack of communication between two voices often leading to messages not being fully understood. Sometimes, a doctor, or a doctor's receptionist, will speak to a patient over the telephone and realise that a home visit is necessary immediately. On other occasions the message is relayed in a confused manner and although the doctor may agree to visit the patient, it may not have been understood that he should do so sooner rather than later on in the day. I think that if patients requesting visits had a better idea of the pattern of work of a doctor, it might well help them to phrase their requests more efficiently.

A doctor's day

The average general practitioner starts his day with a morning surgery and, having finished this, will deal with some routine visits which he has marked in his book on previous days. He will also pick up his share of the new visits in the practice. He may have personally monitored each visit, or he may have left it to his receptionist to note them down. He will try to plan his visiting pattern in the most efficient way, so that he leaves his surgery, drives to his visits and returns to his surgery or home for lunch. If he does not know that a visit is of particular significance, it will be dealt with in a geographical manner rather than because of its medical importance. He may have an afternoon clinic at the local hospital. Alternatively, he may have a late afternoon or early evening surgery, followed by a night on call. Nowadays, most doctors work in group practices, and arrange that each doctor is only on call once or twice a week.

Describing the symptoms

It is important, therefore, when ringing a doctor to make certain that if one uses words like 'collapse', 'stroke', 'heart attack', 'faint', 'unconscious', or 'gasping for breath', one can describe in detail what one means. If the condition is obviously serious the general practitioner will have to stop his morning or afternoon surgery, leave patients in the waiting room and go straight out. This is not something which happens very often, but at times such an action on the part of a doctor can save a patient's life. Every doctor is prepared to abandon surgery and ask his receptionist to explain to the patients that there is a crisis, if it is really necessary.

However, it is somewhat irritating to rush out from surgery, leaving patients in the waiting room, and a succession coming in by appointment, to find that one is not dealing with a heart attack or a stroke but a patient who has felt a little faint, and has not been worried about it, but by chance a near neighbour has called in and panicked.

This sort of thing is part of life in a general practice, but one can imagine that in the middle of a busy winter's day when there is a considerable amount of illness around, this type of false alarm does not lead to good medicine at the time, or possibly during the rest of that morning.

Calling an ambulance

If the general practitioner is not available, or if the illness is thought to be too serious to wait, one can dial 999, ask for the ambulance service and put the problem to them. Almost certainly an ambulance will arrive fairly rapidly and the patient will be transferred to a hospital casualty department. There the matter will be dealt with quickly, and one hopes the condition is sufficiently serious to justify the considerable cost and disruption to the ambulance service involved in taking the patient to hospital.

Basically, casualty departments are present in all large district general hospitals and their function is to deal with accidents and immediate emergencies, being equipped, prepared and very happy to carry out this role. What causes them considerable irritation is when a person arrives late in the evening with a chronic cough, expecting this to be looked at and diagnosed, when in fact he could have been seen by his own doctor during the previous weeks.

Specialist treatment

The vast majority of illnesses are dealt with by the general practitioner, but if he needs it, he has the back up of the technical services, laboratories, x-ray departments and the possibility of referring his patients to a specialist clinic for more detailed advice regarding diagnosis and treatment.

Again, this can lead to conflicts when a patient feels that an early referral is necessary, and the doctor disagrees. I think that over the last few years patients have increasingly accepted that many general practitioners have become more sophisticated in their ability to diagnose and treat, and are not so demanding in their requests for specialist treatment.

If too many patients are referred unnecessarily to specialist clinics, they are bound to get full up, waiting lists will grow, and the patients with the significant problems will have to wait longer to be seen. Whatever criticisms may be levelled against the National Health Service, it still functions in the main in a very efficient manner. However, certain clinics tend to have long waiting lists. In particular, patients normally have to wait a considerable while for appointments with eye, ear, nose and throat, skin or orthopaedic specialists.

The reasons are simple. These particular parts of the body produce many minor and major complaints which need specialised help in diagnosis and treatment. Over the years, money has not been invested in these particular aspects of the National Health Service and therefore patients referred to these clinics have to wait. To relieve this problem, I think that if the condition of a patient on a waiting list improves spontaneously, he should notify his doctor and the clinic, so that his appointment can be given to someone else.

Problems with the specialist

Generally, a doctor is happy to refer a patient to whichever specialist the patient wishes to see, unless he feels that this particular specialist is unsuitable to treat his particular condition. It may be that when the patient has been to a specialist clinic he feels dissatisfied on various counts. Firstly, he may feel irritated that he has not seen the consultant to whom he was referred. Instead, he may have seen an assistant. He feels, therefore, that he did not get the special treatment to which he was entitled. If that is the case, I would suggest that the patient discusses the situation with his doctor. If he agrees with the patient, he may write to the consultant concerned and ask that he will deal with the case personally on the patient's next visit.

Of course, the patient may have seen the consultant, not be prepared to accept his view of the problem, and feel that he needs a further specialist opinion. At times this might be absolutely right, but usually if the general practitioner is good and he has sent the patient to a conscientious specialist, then almost certainly the patient is wrong.

Most general practitioners realise that at times patients find it very difficult to accept that they have a particular disease when they are convinced that they have not, or vice versa. These situations require tact, sympathy and time from the general practitioner in order to try and help the patient. In such circumstances I am usually prepared to arrange for the patient to be seen by one further consultant, but would not recommend multiple referrals in an effort to satisfy the patient that all my colleagues are wrong.

Giving the patient the full facts

One of the problems facing patients and relations is the question of how truthful one's doctor should be. If one feels one is suffering from a life-threatening disorder, should one be told at once or not at all? Should the matter be discussed with one in simple terms, but explored in considerably more detail with one's husband or wife? Should the doctor keep the facts to himself and not discuss them with anyone?

I think that patients are entitled to know what is the matter with them, but that the condition should only be discussed in detail when the doctor is certain of his facts. It seems to me unkind and unnecessary to tell a patient that there is a strong possibility that he may have cancer when one has only a hunch and no positive proof. One can feel very certain that the diagnosis is going to be positive, but it seems to me only fair to wait until one has got a definite answer before opening up the subject for discussion.

If, however, a patient is insistent on knowing the truth at an early stage, he may need to be told and thereafter be involved in the decision-making process, and may well find it an unpleasant situation.

At times the patient is the person who needs to make the decision about medication. It is well known that there is a very small percentage of women who suffer from serious complications when on the pill. If a woman wants protection with no complications, she cannot be placed on oral contraceptives. It is really up to her to make this decision because it is her responsibility to choose her form of contraception. Although I must evaluate the risks, problems and side effects before placing a patient on a specific antibiotic, I do not think this is the case when offering a service to a person who is basically fit. So I leave the choice of the form of contraception to the woman patient. I am very happy, for instance, to prescribe oral contraception. Many of my patients are equally happy to accept it, but if one of them is not, she must accept the final responsibility of whether she wishes to take oral contraceptives, or whether she prefers to use some other form of protection.

Choosing one's treatment

To return to the question of cancer, I do believe that the patient should decide whether he wishes to be involved in heroic forms of surgery or unpleasant forms of medical treatment. A patient has a right to understand the potential hazards to health if the condition is untreated, and equally to be told in detail the immediate and long-term effects of radiation treatment, surgery or chemotherapy. All these treatments can be efficient and effective and produce minimal side effects, but in some cases they can be relatively ineffective, and produce significant deterioration in health and very unpleasant side effects.

In this area of medicine I think the doctor and the patient need to discuss the matter in detail. It is not a question of rights, but the best way to treat someone who is unwell and likely to become worse as the weeks go by.

I should like to finish on a happier note. Most patients, most of the time, get on well with their general practitioners. Over the years, like most of my colleagues, I have had the odd row with a patient, but fortunately at the end of most days I feel that I have enjoyed my work, enjoyed dealing with the potential problems and difficulties which have come my way, and hope that most of my patients have gone away reasonably satisfied. I think this applies to most general practitioners in this country. In spite of the attacks which come our way, I think that most people still feel that their doctor is somebody that they can turn to in times of trouble and crisis, who will offer them a service which they feel is adequate, and that they will be pleased to regard him still as their doctor.

Glossary Of Terms

Absence   Transient loss of consciousness caused by petit mal epilepsy.

Agoraphobia   Fear of open spaces.

Alimentary system   Passage in the body through which food passes, from ingestion to elimination.

Alveoli   Air sacs in the lungs.

Anticholinergic   Drug prescribed in the treatment of Parkinson's disease.

Appendicitis   Inflammation of the appendix.

Bronchitis   Inflammation of the bronchial tubes.

Bronchopneumonia   Scattered patches of pneumonia in the lungs.

Capillary   Tiny blood vessel in which the oxygen and chemicals in the blood diffuse out into the tissue.

Chemotherapy   Use of chemicals in the prevention or treatment of disease.

Chronic   Long-lasting disease.

Claustrophobia   Fear of enclosed spaces.

Cog wheel rigidity   Symptom of Parkinson's disease, when a patient can only bend his joints in a jerky manner.

Convulsion   Involuntary muscle spasm, always accompanied by loss of consciousness.

Deconditioning programme   Method of curing a patient of a phobia.

Denatured   Changed from its original state by the removal of some of its properties.

Disseminated sclerosis   Another name for multiple sclerosis.

Diverticulitis   Inflammation of the diverticula (pockets) in the large intestine.

Dopamine   Chemical substance manufactured in the brain which keeps muscles at the right tension.

Electroencephalogram   (EEG) Highly sophisticated machine which records brain waves.

Emphysema   Condition where there are fewer air sacs in the lungs than normal, with less area in the lungs for the oxygen to diffuse.

Encephalitis lethargica   Inflammation of the brain causing lethargy.

Epilepsy   Condition where disrupted brain activity produces convulsions.

Febrile convulsion   Involuntary muscle spasm and loss of consciousness which occurs in children.

Finger clubbing   Symptom of chronic bronchitis where the ends of the fingers are swollen and nails curved.

Fit   Common term for a convulsion.

Gastro-colic reflex   Nervous reflex, stimulated by a large meal, which signals the desire to empty the bowel.

Grand mal   Major type of epileptic fit.

Haemorrhage   Bleeding.

Haemorrhoids   Group of veins which bulge at the anus, causing discomfort.

Hypoxic   Becoming short of breath due to lack of oxygen in the lungs.

Idiopathic   Disease whose cause is unknown.

Implosion therapy   Method of curing a patient of a phobia.

Laxative   Agent taken to make the bowels open.

Levodopa   Drug which replaces the dopamine not present in the brain of a sufferer of Parkinson's disease.

Lobar pneumonia   Pneumonia confined to one part of the lungs.

Lower respiratory tract infection   Infection of the lungs.

Multiple sclerosis   Disease affecting the nervous pathways in the brain and spinal cord.

Opthalmoscope   Instrument used to examine the eye.

Orthopaedics   Treatment of deformities in bones, muscles, ligaments, joints and tendons.

Petit mal   Minor type of epileptic attack, causing transient loss of consciousness.

Phlebitis   A condition of veins caused by thrombosis forming, usually in the leg.

Infantile convulsion   *See* febrile convulsion.

Phobia   An irrational fear or panic caused by a certain object or situation.

Physiotherapy   Treatment of disease by the use of physical methods such as heat, exercise, massage and manipulation.

Pill rolling   Uncontrollable movement of the hands, present in Parkinson's disease.

Plasma   The blood minus the red and white cells.

Pneumonia   Infection of the fine lung tissue.

Pre frontal leucotomy   Operation performed on the front of the brain, to cure extreme cases of phobias.

Secondary epilepsy   Epilepsy caused by problems at birth, or disease or accidents later in life.

Sputum   Mucous material coughed up from the lungs.

Substantia nigra   Portion of the brain, so-called because of its dark pigmentation.

Swamping therapy   *See* implosion therapy.

Temporal lobe epilepsy   Condition giving localised involuntary movement, such as lip smacking.

Thrombosis   A blood clot which forms in a blood vessel.

Upper respiratory tract infection   Infection of the mouth, nose or throat.

Varicose eczema   Skin which is thin and discoloured at the site of a varicose vein.

Venous system   System of veins within the body.

Useful Addresses

Action on Smoking and Health (ASH)
27-35 Mortimer Street
London W1N 7RJ
Tel: 01-637 9843

Age Concern
Bernard Sunley House
60 Pitcairn Road
Mitcham
Surrey CR4 3LL
Tel: 01-640 5431

British Epilepsy Association
Crowthorne House
New Wokingham Road
Wokingham
Berkshire RG11 3AY
Tel: Wokingham 463122

The British Nutrition Foundation
15 Belgrave Square
London SW1
Tel: 01-235 4904

Send sae for advice on nutrition and general health

The Chest, Heart and Stroke Association
Tavistock House North
Tavistock Square
London WC1H 9JE
Tel: 01-387 3012

Disabled Living Foundation
346 Kensington High Street
London W14 8NS
Tel: 01-602 2491

Health Education Council
78 New Oxford Street
London WC1A 1AH
Tel: 01-637 1881

Mental Health Foundation
10 Hallam Street
London W1N 6DH
Tel: 01-580 0145

Multiple Sclerosis Society
286 Munster Road
London SW6 6AP
Tel: 01-381 4022

National Association for Mental Health (MIND)
22 Harley Street
London W1N 2ED
Tel: 01-637 0741

Parkinson's Disease Society of the UK Ltd
81 Queens Road
London SW19 8NR
Tel: 01-946 2500

Patients Association
11 Dartmouth Street
London SW1
Tel: 01-222 4992

The Phobics Society
4 Cheltenham Road
Chorlton-cum-Hardy
Manchester M21 1QN
Tel: Manchester 881 1937

Psychiatric Rehabilitation Association
21a Kingsland High Street
London E8
Tel: 01-254 9753

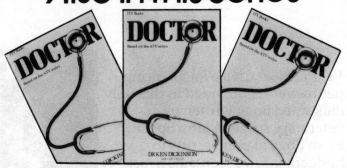

Also In This Series

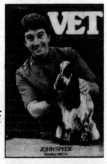

Vet Practical advice for all caring pet-owners is provided in this fully illustrated book written by veterinary surgeon John Speer. From dogs to ponies, cats to budgerigars, Vet contains a mass of information on selection, handling and care of most household pets. £1.50

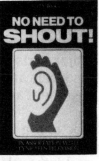

No Need To Shout Written by experts, this book is aimed not only at coping with hearing difficulties, but families and friends in contact with the hard of hearing. £1.50

Learn To Sing This helpful book, written by writer, singer and teacher Graham Hewitt, provides a wealth of practical advice to help improve your singing ability and general vocal skills. £1

Home Made For The Home (Book 2) This fully illustrated book gives many ideas and clear step by step instructions on how to use a variety of skills and crafts to enable you to make attractive and useful articles for the home, in the home. £1

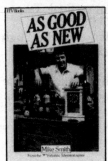

Further copies of this book are available from:

Doctor Book Two
PO Box 50
Market Harborough
Leicestershire

Cheques/PO's made payable to ITV Books
price £1.50 (including postage and packing)

ITV Books, Competition House, Farndon Road, Market Harborough, Leicestershire